Praise for *Duty*

"One can easily be impressed by the accolades and awards that a person has gathered through the years. I am certainly fascinated by Dr. Novello's accomplishments and trajectory from Puerto Rico to United States Surgeon General. But what truly touches my heart and deeply impresses me is to see how a human being cares for another human being in a time of need. . . . I was mesmerized to see Dr. Toni Novello taking care of her former husband, Dr. Joe Novello, as he was battling brain cancer. . . . Thank you, Toni, for giving me this gift to witness the beauty of humanity. Reading this book allows me to dream of a better world."

—**Dr. Q, Alfredo Quiñones-Hinojosa**, MD, FAANS, FACS,
William J. and Charles H. Mayo Professor,
Monica Flynn Jacoby Endowed Chair, Neurologic Surgery Chair,
James C. and Sarah K. Kennedy Dean of Research, Mayo Clinic

"*Duty Calls* demonstrates that Dr. Antonia Novello's legacy of leadership is built upon her unwavering commitment to serve those in need, regardless of her position or title. Her actions during Hurricane Maria in Puerto Rico stand as a testament to her tenacity and ability to motivate and mobilize those around her. . . ."

—**Maria Fernanda Levis-Peralta**, MPH, MPA, PCMH-CCE,
CEO, Impactivo Consulting

"*Duty Calls* underscores Dr. Novello's strong character, high principles, and extraordinary compassion. . . . She is a champion of the underprivileged, sympathetic to the needs of all Americans, a sensitive and diplomatic public servant. She was successful because she did not care who got the credit, so long as the proper thing was done."

—**Rabbi Abraham Blum**, New York State Chaplain;
Chief, Westchester County Chaplain Office; Special Assistant,
Commissioner of the Department of Correction, State of New York;
Advisory Committee, Central Rabbinical Congress of
the United States and Canada

"A rare trailblazer in the world of public health, Dr. Antonia Novello's life of commitment and public service, as documented in *Duty Calls*, is nothing short of groundbreaking and inspirational."

—**Chanie Sternberg**, President/CEO, Refuah Health Center

"My respect and admiration for Dr. Novello, which began when she was working on her doctorate at Johns Hopkins University, has been amplified by reading about the many obstacles she has overcome during her life and career. I was inspired by *Duty Calls*—and you will be, too!"

—**Alfred Sommer**, MD, Dean Emeritus, Professor Emeritus, Bloomberg School of Public Health, Johns Hopkins University

"Congresswoman Shirley Chisholm said, 'Service is the rent you pay for living.' Service has defined Dr. Novello's life and career, as she writes in *Duty Calls*. It is a must-read book for every leader, novice or experienced, wanting to learn what public service is all about."

—**Major General Jose J. Reyes**, Adjutant General, National Guard, Puerto Rico

"Dr. Novello's service as a humanitarian has been memorialized through the Dr. Antonia Novello Humanitarian Medallion of the United States Hispanic Leadership Institute. I am so indebted to her for saving my life, and I am thrilled to recommend her book for all to understand how she embodies humanitarianism of the highest order."

—**Juan Andrade**, President, United States Hispanic Leadership Institute

"I was privileged to witness Dr. Novello perform admirably as a humble servant when no one was looking and there was very little to be gained. How someone performs in these circumstances reveals their true character and greatness. I hope you will read and be inspired by the story of this remarkable woman!"

—**Robert Paeglow**, MD, Founder, President, and Medical Director, Koinonia Primary Care

"How fascinating to read *Duty Calls* to find out the real story of this outstanding Puerto Rican pediatrician and leader in the health-care industry."
—**Norman Maldonado**, MD, Chancellor, Medical Campus of the University of Puerto Rico; President, University of Puerto Rico, 1993–2001

"As Dr. Novello's patient at the University of Michigan in the early 1970s, I so admire her dedication, commitment, and drive that come through so clearly in *Duty Calls*."
—**Patrick Roush**, President and Creative Director, Roush Specialty Services

"Dr. Novello's commitment to public service is evidenced clearly in *Duty Calls*, along with many anecdotes that will delight its readers for their uniqueness and wisdom."
—**Sila M. Calderón**, Chief of Staff to the Governor of Puerto Rico, 1985–1990; Secretary of State [Puerto Rico], 1988–1990; Mayor of San Juan, 1997–2000; Governor of Puerto Rico, 2001–2004; Chair of the Board of the Center of Puerto Rico/Sila M. Calderón Foundation

"Since [Dr. Novello] was the first woman and first Hispanic to become Surgeon General of the United States, this book is long overdue. Dr. Novello has proven that she cares about medicine, public health, and America. In *Duty Calls*, this outstanding physician, scientist, and public health leader demonstrates clearly her commitment to service and the health of all members of the public. The reader will be informed and inspired."
—**David Satcher**, MD, PhD, 16th Surgeon General of the United States; 10th Assistant Secretary for Health in the Department of Health and Human Services; former Director of the Centers for Disease Control; Administrator of the Agency for Toxic Substances and Disease Registry; and Founding Director and Senior Advisor, Satcher Health Leadership Institute, Morehouse School of Medicine

"This is a deeply personal story that lays it all out, both good and bad. Through her frank revelation, we are allowed to see into the heart and mind of a truly remarkable woman, physician, and public servant. It's not just a story of glamorous achievements and recognitions, but a story that, page by page, shows us the essence of a life well lived through all its challenges, obstacles, tragedy, and high-level achievements. . . . At its core, this book focuses on the guiding life principles and heart of the author. . . . Thank you, Antonia, for helping us learn from you as we also strive to be better servants and live meaningful, purpose-filled lives."

—**John Zubialde**, MD, Executive Dean, College of Medicine, University of Oklahoma Health Sciences Center

"*Duty Calls* is an inspiring book about the challenges, triumphs, and historic achievements of The Honorable Dr. Antonia Novello, the nation's first woman and first Hispanic US Surgeon General. . . . Dr. Novello is a nationally renowned and award-winning leader who never forgot her Hispanic and Puerto Rican roots. Reading her book will remind all of us that even when life deals us challenging and unexpected curveballs, we can still overcome and achieve success to our highest potential. . . . Dr. Novello's memoir will inspire you as it inspired me."

—**Cid Wilson**, President and CEO, Hispanic Association on Corporate Responsibility

"Dr. Novello's dedication, compassion, kindness, sacrifice, and service to the needy and to her country are on full display in *Duty Calls*. She uses her intellectual capacity to its utmost, goes out of her way to help after natural disasters and during emergencies, and has never forgotten her roots throughout her life. This book tells the story of the wonderful woman I know who carries with her the noblest feelings that human beings can possess."

—**Dr. Aida Diaz**, Past President, Puerto Rico Teachers Association

"Through her exemplary life of service, Dr. Novello has answered to the highest call of duty: be at the service of others. As Surgeon General, she was instrumental in advocating for those more marginalized by the public health system. And during Puerto Rico's disastrous experience with Hurricane María, Dr. Novello's leadership and selflessness brought quick-needed relief when and where it was most needed. Her inspirational life as documented in *Duty Calls* is truly a life well lived."

—**Luis A. Ferré Rangel**, President of the Board,
Centros Sor Isolina Ferré Puerto Rico

"*Duty Calls* from Dr. Antonia Novello, the first woman and first Hispanic US Surgeon General, takes readers on an autobiographical journey from her childhood through adulthood. She details the world of medicine, her service to others, and the life lessons she has learned along the way. Nothing is left out—the good and the bad of an extraordinary life."

—**Yocasta Brugal**, MD, President, CEO, and Dean, San Juan Bautista
School of Medicine; forensic and anatomic pathologist

"This book is a powerful reminder of the importance of knowing and owning your space as a leader. Dr. Novello offers insightful advice that will resonate with leaders across the entire continuum of their careers. . . . I was struck by the dedication to excellence and uncompromising standards she possesses and how [they] show up in her work and personal pursuits. . . . She exemplifies a true servant leader! . . . Phenomenal read."

—**Rear Admiral (retired) Sylvia Trent-Adams**, PhD, RN, President,
University of North Texas Health Science Center at Fort Worth

"There are moments when the best of humankind comes forward unexpectedly, and then there are moments when humankind is not acknowledged or recognized [for] doing the best of work, in silence, constantly delivering care for those in need. Dr. Novello is that special person as demonstrated in her memoir, *Duty Calls*. After Hurricane Maria, Dr. Novello found a way to provide health care to many. We will honor her many selfless acts of service when our emergency room and acute care clinic are finished, by naming our clinic in Dr. Novello's honor. Her life of service has benefited so many, and her memoir will inspire countless others."

—**Tito Valentin**, community activist and President, COSSAO (Corporation
of Primary Health Services and Socio-Economic Development)

"...A compelling memoir of a remarkable physician and pediatric nephrologist, and the first woman and first Hispanic US Surgeon General.... The story of her life dedicated to serving others, overcoming all kinds of difficulties, and leading by example will inspire readers to challenge the status quo and embrace their potential to create a better, more equitable world for all."

—**Juan Carlos Caicedo**, MD.FACS; Professor of Surgery; Surgical Director, Liver Transplant Program; Director, Living Donor Liver Transplant and Hepatobiliary Program; Director, Hispanic Transplant Program; Transplant Surgeon, Northwestern Memorial Hospital; Pediatric Transplant Surgeon, Lurie Children's Hospital, Northwestern Medicine

"Dr. Antonia Novello tells the story of her life—medical challenges, professional successes, painful losses, and power at the highest level—all in one nonstop narrative of love and betrayal and bravery. Her story is as much about pain as it is about triumph, but it is mostly about one little sick girl who turns into one powerful medical visionary. My favorite advice from Dr. Novello is this: 'I only wish I had spent more time loving, less time judging. More hugging, rather than distancing which I did to protect myself from pain.' Read *Duty Calls* to discover how to do more hugging and loving, lessons worthy of her amazing life."

—**Timothy Shriver**, Chairman, Special Olympics

"This book . . . is going to challenge you, inspire you, and move you to tears. It is the story of a remarkable woman who dared to speak her mind and use the truth as a weapon to help the most underprivileged. . . . It is an invaluable source where you will get the opportunity to know the story of one of the most influential women of our time told in her own words."

—**Dr. Gustavo Laabes**, Primary Care Volunteer Physician, Beige Caps Founder

Duty Calls

Duty Calls

Lessons Learned from
an Unexpected Life of Service

Antonia Coello Novello, MD, MPH, DrPH
with Jill S. Tietjen, PE

Fulcrum Publishing
Wheat Ridge, Colorado

Library of Congress Cataloging-in-Publication Data
Names: Novello, Antonia C., author. | Tietjen, Jill S., author.
Title: Duty calls : lessons learned from an unexpected life of service /
    Antonia C. Novello, M.D. with Jill S. Tietjen, P.E.
Description: Wheat Ridge, Colorado : Fulcrum Publishing, [2024]
Identifiers: LCCN 2023039973 (print) | LCCN 2023039974 (ebook) | ISBN
    9781682754467 (paperback) | ISBN 9781682754474 (ebook)
Subjects: LCSH: Novello, Antonia C. | Health officers--United
    States--Biography. | Pediatricians--United States--Biography. | Women
    pediatricians--United States--Biography. | Hispanic American
    pediatricians--Biography. | BISAC: BIOGRAPHY & AUTOBIOGRAPHY / Political
    | BIOGRAPHY & AUTOBIOGRAPHY / Personal Memoirs
Classification: LCC R154.N82 A3 2024 (print) | LCC R154.N82 (ebook) | DDC
    618.9200092 [B]--dc23/eng/20231107
LC record available at https://lccn.loc.gov/2023039973
LC ebook record available at https://lccn.loc.gov/2023039974

Unless otherwise noted, all photos are from the
private collection of Dr. Antonia C. Novello.
Photo on p. 102 courtesy of Society of Education and
Rehabilitation of Puerto Rico (SER de PR).
Photo on p. 129 courtesy of Johns Hopkins Bloomberg School of Public Health.

Cover design by Kateri Kramer

Printed in the United States
0 9 8 7 6 5 4 3 2 1

Fulcrum Publishing
3970 Youngfield Street
Wheat Ridge, Colorado 80033
(800) 992-2908 • (303) 277-1623
www.fulcrumbooks.com

To my mother,
Ana Delia Flores, who shaped me with her love
and high expectations.

To my former husband, Dr. Joseph R. Novello,
who through his actions—for better or worse—pulled me out
of an average life and helped me thrive in a new one.

To Jill,
who inspired me and translated through her words
the reality of my life.

To Nora,
who gave so much to all
and expected nothing in return.

To Marcia and Michael,
who gave me shelter when I needed it the most.

To Mami Loli,
who always cared for
and watched over me.

To Lydia and Yolly,
thank you for always being there for me.

To Dr. Josel Szepsenwol (Chepi),
who sent me to the Mayo Clinic and to whom
I will be forever grateful.

To Dr. Markham Anderson,
who saved my life at the Mayo Clinic
and who believed in me.

Contents

Foreword by The Honorable George E. Pataki,
   53rd Governor of the State of New York...*xv*
Foreword by Jeffrey S. Buchanan,
   Lieutenant General, US Army (Retired)..*xvii*
Co-Author's Note...*xix*
Preface...*xxi*
January 26, 2009..*xxiii*

Part I

Chapter 1. Eighteen Years of Constipation and Consternation 3
Chapter 2. A Kindly Professor and the Mayo Clinic Saved My Life.......... 20
Chapter 3. Destiny and Marriage 41
Chapter 4. Off to Michigan 50
Chapter 5. Washington, D.C., Beckons 62

Part II

Chapter 6. The Pediatrician of the Nation.. 80
Chapter 7. UNICEF and Beyond.. 119
Chapter 8. So Much More Than Vaccines 130
Chapter 9. Framed by the Albany 5 163
Chapter 10. Duty Still Calls.. 173
Epilogue... 203
Life Lessons and Rules to Live By.. 205

Afterword by Nilda Morales,
    President and CEO, Society of Education and
    Rehabilitation of Puerto Rico 211
Afterword by James J. Barba, JD,
    President Emeritus, Albany Medical Center 215

Acknowledgments.. *221*
Awards and Honors.. *223*
Discussion Questions *241*
About the Authors... *243*

Foreword

The Honorable George E. Pataki,
53rd Governor of the State of New York

While I had many great people helping me during my successful twelve years and three terms as Governor of New York State, I
must say that one of the best decisions I made during that time was
appointing Dr. Antonia Novello as my Commissioner of Health.

Health care had emerged as a major issue during my terms,
particularly dealing with the uninsured. Well before the Affordable
Care Act, Dr. Novello and I devised a comprehensive plan to create
new market-based programs without raising taxes that would allow
affordable health insurance to be available for the millions of previously uninsured New Yorkers. Together, we created several new
programs, including Family Health Plus, Child Health Plus, and
Healthy New York. These initiatives were enormously successful and
affordable; comprehensive health care became available for virtually
every resident of New York State.

During my time as Governor, we also faced numerous crises,
including the West Nile and SARS viruses. The most significant crisis was the unforgettable terrorist attacks of September 11, 2001. We
suffered horrific loss of human life, devastating economic disrup-
tion, and a very real health crisis. In addition to the consequences
of the attacks, in New York we also had the crisis of the release of
deadly anthrax, which was discovered in several offices, from media
to government buildings to hospitals. Of course, we also had to deal

with the consequences of tens of thousands of people being exposed to the toxic air at Ground Zero.

Dr. Novello took the key leadership role in ensuring that we responded aggressively and successfully to the anthrax crisis, and that we worked to make sure a comprehensive program was in place to deal with those who were ill as a result of their time at Ground Zero. For this, she was deservedly awarded recognition by the National Governors Association for the outstanding leadership and service she provided during September 11.

Throughout her time as Health Commissioner, Dr. Novello made it a priority to increase access to health care for underserved communities, particularly Latino communities in New York State. She and I were able to visit and expand offerings to what had previously been dramatically underserved communities, including Puerto Ricans, Dominicans, Mexicans, Colombians, and numerous other residents. Together, we were able to put in place programs to make sure that they had access to adequate health care like other New Yorkers, and to ensure that those services were provided by community-based organizations knowledgeable of the unique needs of the diverse populations they served.

I cannot tell you enough how important the leadership of Dr. Novello was. We worked hand in hand for her entire term as Health Commissioner, and in the process, we provided dramatically improved and more affordable health care to all New Yorkers. I am honored to have had her as my Health Commissioner for six years, and I am honored to have the privilege of writing this foreword to her memoir, *Duty Calls*.

Thank you, Dr. Novello, for your life of service.

Foreword

Jeffrey S. Buchanan,
Lieutenant General, US Army (Retired)

I first met Dr. Antonia Novello in the fall of 2017 after Hurricane Maria devastated the island of Puerto Rico. We were both there to help desperate people in their time of greatest need. About a week after the hurricane's landfall, I had been directed to fly to the island and assume command of all the military forces supporting the Federal Emergency Management Agency (FEMA) and the Commonwealth of Puerto Rico. Our response force was very capable and included four ships, seventy-two helicopters, three large and five small expeditionary hospitals, and about fifteen thousand troops. In contrast, Dr. Novello made her own way to the island as a volunteer. She did not have the vast resources that I controlled; all she had was herself. Antonia leveraged her experience, reputation, and her unshakable tenacity to do everything she could for her fellow Puerto Ricans. She had an incredibly positive impact everywhere she went. When she asked for help, I gave her all that I could—and she used it to great effect. We will never know the metrics, but Dr. Novello saved hundreds of lives. Just as importantly, she raised spirits and inspired all to excel.

If you ask your typical American who their heroes are, you'll get the names of movie stars, professional athletes, famous musicians, and even internet "influencers." Unfortunately, we have confused celebrity status with heroism. The word "hero" comes from the ancient Greeks. There are only two requirements to become a hero: courageous acts and a noble purpose. Being a hero is not about being rich, talented, beautiful, or famous, it is about the choices one makes. Dr. Antonia Novello is one of my heroes, and she will be one of yours as well.

Duty Calls is a great memoir because it is not just a historical record of a life, but rather a collection of stories that inspires us all to become better versions of ourselves. Throughout her life, Dr. Novello has faced adversity . . . and persevered. She overcame the effects of a debilitating childhood disease and a botched surgery to excel in medical school, internship, and residency. She overcame the effects of an unfaithful husband and divorce to care for that ex-husband and his family on their deathbeds. She overcame all the doubters and naysayers and rose to become the 14th Surgeon General of the United States, and then employed that office to fight the AIDS epidemic and childhood addictions. In the wake of 9/11, Dr. Novello overcame institutional resistance to get hospitals and emergency rooms the supplies and equipment they needed to care for the thousands of victims. In retirement, she overcame allegations of impropriety stemming from her service as the Health Commissioner of New York. The consistent theme through all this adversity is Dr. Novello's courage to persevere and her steadfast devotion to serving others. Courageous acts and a noble purpose. She is a true American hero. I hope that you are as inspired by her story as I am.

Co-Author's Note

I first met Dr. Antonia Novello in Seneca Falls, New York, in 1994. She was being inducted into the National Women's Hall of Fame, and I was the acceptor for my nominee, Admiral Grace Murray Hopper. I was so impressed by Dr. Novello's charisma and what she said. I thought at the time that if she ever ran for President of the United States, I would drop everything I was doing and work on her campaign.

Over the years, I saw her again at inductions in Seneca Falls, and one year is particularly memorable to me. We were standing outside under a reception tent. Dr. Novello was in a beautiful white suit; I was holding a glass of red punch. She said to keep my glass of punch far away from her! I did so.

In 2014, I was President of the Board of Directors of the National Women's Hall of Fame. The National Hall held a joint panel discussion with the Florida Women's Hall of Fame in Boca Raton, Florida. Dr. Novello was on the panel, and I learned more of her story and the obstacles she had overcome during her life's journey.

In December 2021, I needed endorsements for my book *Over, Under, Around, and Through: How Hall of Famers Surmount Obstacles*. I decided to go very far out on a limb and ask her for her endorsement. The email address I had for her no longer worked, so I sent her a message with my request to connect with her on LinkedIn. She responded immediately, and I got an endorsement. It turned out that Dr. Novello had an item on her bucket list, and she thought I could help: she wanted to get her book published. She was right, I could help. Not only did I help her find a publisher, as fate would have it, I ended up as her co-author.

Life has so many interesting twists and turns. Thirty years after we first met, her book is being published, a book that I have been privileged to be associated with. It dovetails with Dr. Novello's saying, "Preparation meets opportunity," and my philosophy "that you have to keep your eyes open and take advantage of the opportunities that come your way."

I am proud to tell women's stories and delighted that we were able to work together on this important book.

Jill S. Tietjen, PE

Preface

Why this book? Why now? Well, I'm not getting any younger, and I want this to be written while I still remember. But there is so much more.

I haven't told my story. I'm currently one of the few US Surgeons General without a book. There isn't an endowed chair of medicine or pediatrics or public health at a university in my name either. Why? The first female US Surgeon General and the first Hispanic US Surgeon General. Shouldn't there be? Maybe it is because the Latin population is so diverse, without a leader to carry all of us whether we are Mexican, Puerto Rican, Central American, South American, Cuban, or Dominican.

I want young Latinas to know that it is possible to start with a normal background, and then through education and hard work achieve their dreams and still be close and loving with their friends and family. I'm from a middle-sized town in Puerto Rico. My mother, stepfather, and brother were my family. Our family wasn't rich, but we weren't poor, either. My mother was a teacher and school principal. I had a good education but not at a mainland university. Education was crucial. You don't have to be golden to be number one, you just need the desire to go beyond what you are today. And it is okay if it takes you longer to graduate from college than other students. Most Latinos finish college in six years rather than four because they also usually work

> "You don't have to be golden to be number one, you just need the desire to go beyond what you are today."

thirty hours a week. Many also attend local colleges because of their parents' desire to keep them close to the nest.

> "You must decide what legacy you want to leave."

You must decide what legacy you want to leave. I continued my education, thus, I was prepared, and preparation successfully met opportunity, which equaled success. Do the job that nobody else wants to do and do it well. Underpromise and overdeliver. Pick your battles carefully. Surprise wins the war.

I was born in Fajardo, Puerto Rico, with a disease (congenital megacolon or Hirschsprung's disease) that caused me to be hospitalized for two weeks every summer until I was eighteen. Congenital megacolon can occur in combination with other conditions including Down's syndrome or deafness. I feel that God spared me and just had me suffer from extreme constipation because there were bigger plans for my life.

> "Nothing is impossible if you really want to get there. Keep going. Trust your gut. Don't let anybody hold you back."

But those bigger plans were not obvious when I was young. Despite my constipation and hospital stays, my mother would not let me feel sorry for myself. She had high expectations for me. Yet there isn't anybody, including me, who thought I would be Surgeon General of the United States or Health Commissioner of the State of New York during September 11.

I made it despite the odds. It wasn't easy, and I have the scars to prove it. Being first is never easy. I intended to be a good role model, always doing the right thing. Nothing is impossible if you really want to get there. Keep going. Trust your gut. Don't let anybody hold you back. After reading this book, you will see that if I could do it, so can you.

Antonia Coello Novello, MD, MPH, DrPH,
14th United States Surgeon General

January 26, 2009

Am I going to jail? The phone rang at six thirty in the morning. In my life experience, early morning phone calls are generally harbingers of bad news. It was my niece calling from Puerto Rico. I expected bad news about my mother. My niece was crying, hysterical, saying over and over, "Titi, tell me that it isn't true." I asked her what she was talking about. It obviously wasn't about my mother. She told me the front page of both the *New York Times* and the Puerto Rican newspaper said I had been accused of multiple counts, including felonies, and that I faced probable jail time. That these charges stemmed from my tenure as Commissioner of the Department of Health of the State of New York. I was stunned. What was happening to me, the little girl from Fajardo, Puerto Rico, and why now, two years after I had left that office?

Part I

Everyone's life encompasses a series of challenges; mine felt especially daunting, a combination of cultural, gender-related, and health issues that all conspired to hold me back. And yet, I was able to persevere and find the opportunities hidden in all of these challenges.

CHAPTER 1

Eighteen Years of Constipation and Consternation

I was born in my grandmother's house in Fajardo, Puerto Rico, on August 23, 1944. My grandmother (Paula Santana) was a very strong-willed woman. She had two different birthdates so she could always get two sets of presents and have two parties all in the same year. It does not surprise me then that my mother married young. My father, according to my mother, was a very handsome policeman, quite a bit older than she. When they married, they moved to his hometown, Jayuya, in the center of the island of Puerto Rico, where my mother continued her career as a teacher.

At the time of my birth, you had to be born in the presence of your grandmother because she would then babysit and otherwise tend to you and your mother. My parents had traveled to my grandmother's house in Fajardo from Jayuya because there was no arguing with Mamá—this was how and where I, her first grandchild, was going to be born. My grandmother, Mamá, as we called her, arranged for the midwife, who was present at my birth. It was the same midwife who had been present at the births of my mother, her four half sisters, and almost all the people in the neighborhood.

I was named Antonia after my father, Antonio Coello. He wanted a boy, so I was stuck with a derivative of his name. I understand that I look very much like him, but I don't remember him because my parents divorced when I was quite young. My brother, Tomas, was born in

June 1946. Our half brother, Martin, whose mother was our maid, was born in October 1946. The birth of my half brother, and our father's relationship with the maid, led Mami—as I called my mother (Ana Delia Flores)—to leave our father that December when I was two years old and Tomas was still an infant. She told our father: "Take a good look at your children, because you will never see them again." And he never did. I know that my mother did not have a happy marriage with my father, as she used to talk to me about it when I was older. He died when I was in seventh grade, but I felt nothing when I learned of his death. I never referred to him as Dad—or Father. Mami also refused to allow anyone in her family to have contact with him.

Mami would not brook any dissent with her edict of no contact with my father, including from her four half sisters. When I graduated from first grade, my maternal aunts took a picture of me and were planning to mail it to my father. I was dressed all in white, I had my diploma, and I think at that time I looked very much like him. Somehow my mother found out about their plan, and the next day, as we were all watching the corner mailbox in anticipation of the mailman, there was my mother, standing and waiting. I guess she asked to see all the letters that came out of that mailbox. When she found the one sent by my aunts, she looked at all of us across the street from her as she ripped it into pieces and threw it away. Never again did my aunts fail to heed my mother's requests.

After she left my father, Mami moved back to her mother's house. What else really could she do? A single woman in a little town with two children and no job. She started teaching night school to make ends meet and to help Mamá, who worked in the school cafeteria. Mamá was still raising my four aunts, the oldest of whom had just entered high school. Mami did not last long living under her mother's roof.

Mami married one of her night-school pupils a few years later. He was the only father I really knew, and they were married for fifty-five years. His name was Ramon Rosario, and he was called

"Moncho." He was an electrician and a very kind man, and he met all the needs that I had for a father. Mami told him from the first date that these were her children and that she was responsible for them. "You can correct them, but they are mine."

> "And when you challenge me, I am going to prove you wrong no matter how long it takes. It is part of my DNA."

My maternal aunt Dolores was my favorite aunt; I used to call her Mami Loli. She was a nurse and she tended to me always. Not only was she there through all my childhood diseases, but she also took me to the hospital where she worked and told the doctors, "This is my niece, and she wants to become a doctor." The doctors all laughed. I was ten, and I took that laughter as a challenge. And when you challenge me, I am going to prove you wrong no matter how long it takes. It is part of my DNA. Some people do things they are told they can – I do things I was told I could not.

Those doctors were just reflecting the culture of Puerto Rico at the time. To be a girl in Puerto Rico in the 1950s and 1960s usually meant that your parents insisted that you stay on the island. They probably didn't even want you in the continental United States if you were married. You were supervised or you had a curfew—or worse, you had a chaperone present during your dates.

* * *

Because I was born with a condition called congenital megacolon (also called Hirschsprung's disease), I was physically different from the other children. This is a disease where you are missing nerve cells in the large intestine. As a result, you don't have regular bowel movements. The cellular plexus (Auerbach plexus) that moves the intestines was missing for several feet, meaning that I suffered from chronic constipation.

My belly would get bigger and bigger until enemas, with a variety of different additives, were administered, and then I would have a flat belly. All the while growing up, the condition with the big belly and constant constipation was mostly tolerable because everyone in my hometown knew about it and its causes and effects. In addition to the weekly enemas, each summer I would spend two weeks in the hospital being cleaned out. I wanted to be a medical doctor because I was inspired by the way in which the nurses cared for me and gave me hope.

For some people, like the Carpenters' song said, rainy days and Mondays were difficult days. Not for me. It wasn't rainy days and Mondays—it was Saturdays. I hated Saturdays. When I walked into the kitchen and saw the pot of water boiling (with a pinch of salt), I knew what came next. I was getting enemas to clean out my bowels. The enemas were administered by Eliza, our maid Juana's daughter. Because there were no hooks on the bathroom wall, she had to hold the enema bag high for the water to run down to my intestine. There were many enemas that day—sometimes five or ten—until Mami was convinced that my bowels were clean. I was held hostage in the bathroom for hours, alone and feeling sorry for myself. I'm sure the rest of my family hated Saturdays as well—they couldn't use our bathroom for all those hours.

Mami was always on the hunt for more effective enemas. Thus, whenever I saw her talking to the neighbors, I dreaded what was coming next. They were almost always discussing the newest enema fad—something more powerful than the standard saline enema. And we just had to try it.

One particularly memorable episode was the hydrogen peroxide enema (I still don't know who offered this advice). Oh, my goodness, did it burn! And it didn't help. But I am convinced that if something happens to me and I can't be identified by outward physical characteristics, someone just needs to open up my intestines and they'll know it's me—because they will be blond.

Mami was empathetic about my medical condition, but she wasn't sympathetic. I was not going to get away with murder because of my congenital megacolon. I went to school. I studied. Education was important. When I needed something, she ensured that I got it. All the things I wanted she would buy for me. She was never going to allow the disease to stop me, and neither was I. I would come home from school and immediately work on my assignments. You might say I was obsessed. Some of my classmates would copy my answers, never doing their own work. I was always at home studying. I could have breaks if I completed my studying—then I could have fun. Everything had to be earned. You want to go to the plaza and be with your friends on Saturday? You have to do the bathrooms on Saturday morning. Or you have to babysit your cousins. There was always quid pro quo.

All my life, I utilized humor and hidden intelligence to bypass my medical issues. No one pays attention to the joker. They assume that your intelligence is zero when you are the joker. And I was not ever going to let any negative comments about my intelligence or my intestinal problem deter me from what I wanted to accomplish. There were already enough impediments in my way—I didn't need any more.

When I was eleven or twelve years old, I had not gone to the bathroom in a while, but I lied to Mami and said I had. Yet I knew I was in trouble because my belly was large and hard. Every trick in the book got used—Milk of Magnesia, castor oil, soapy enemas with Castile soap—nothing happened. Apparently, I had not fooled Mami. She had arranged for me to go to the hospital to have my stools extracted manually. This was a desperation maneuver that I did not know was in the offing.

The night before I was to go to the hospital, Mami arranged for a woman known as the *santiguera*, a healer who specialized in abdominal discomfort, to come and do her technique on me. The *santiguera* put warm oil on my belly and then started rubbing. Up, down, clockwise, counterclockwise, all the while, pushing my belly in every possible direction and pushing down with force, especially on my left side. After she was finished, I was exhausted and went to bed. I knew I was due at the hospital the next day, but I still didn't know what for.

I woke up the next morning, and to my surprise I had the desire to go to the bathroom naturally—without an enema—so I went. I didn't go into the toilet—I was so desperate that I squatted on the floor in front of the bathtub. I was there a long time. When it was over, there was a mountain of stool—about twelve inches tall and six inches wide. Even though I was feeling very weak, I called Mami and saw the amazement on her face. Possibly, she was relieved that now I wouldn't have to go to the hospital for manual extractions. It was such an event that the whole neighborhood came to see my success. I was so tired, I paid little attention. Mami gave me a glass of hot milk and I went to bed.

I must confess I hardly ate anything for a week after that. I was petrified of getting a big belly again. Obviously, that couldn't go on forever and was short-lived. The entire experience taught me not to lie to my mother again regarding my bathroom routine.

* * *

Despite my disease, most of my youth was spent in the normal activities that children pursue. For me, Girl Scouting was formative. I remember going to Mami saying, "Mami, I need five dollars because I am joining the Brownies." This is when I was in third grade. Mami just gave me the money. I joined the troop, and I think that was the best thing that ever happened in my youth because it put me in groups. It put me into competitiveness. And it helped me see how you can make it even if you are an average child in an average neighborhood with an average everything. I became very competitive, and my troop leader became my godmother for my Catholic confirmation.

After being a Brownie, I was a Girl Scout—all the way through high school. I stopped being a Girl Scout my first year of college when they wouldn't let me sell cookies in the student lounge. That was the end of my Girl Scout career. By then, I had earned so many badges that between them and the ribbons, I looked like a very well-decorated war veteran or a flying nun!

I used to go to Girl Scout camp one week every summer, first as a Girl Scout and then as a camp counselor (I was assigned six girls). I always took the upper bunk bed because for the longest time, I had bad experiences with bed wetters when I was in the lower bunk.

There were plays, games, and opportunities to get ribbons. With my competitive spirit, I had to participate, as always. On one occasion, ribbons were being awarded for table setting under water.

This was the way it worked. You had to dive into the pool and find the plate, the fork, the knife, the spoon, and the glass. You then brought all the pieces to the deck of the pool and set the table. I was able to gather all the pieces perfectly as I dove into the pool. I got every piece I needed before anybody else. However, I almost lost my ribbon because I had never been told where the utensils went around the plate. I was in agony thinking I had almost drowned—which was now all in vain—until the lifeguard gave me some hints and I set the table and won the ribbon.

Never underestimate a girl from Fajardo. We weren't called the Hard Faces (Cariduros) for no reason!

During my scouting years, the College of Lawyers (the Puerto Rican Bar Association) held a poetry contest. My godmother (my Girl Scout leader) and I attended to watch another Girl Scout enact a poem. She used many hand gestures and completed her turn. My godmother said, "Why don't you recite a poem, too?" So, unprepared, but familiar with the poem, I got up and gave the same poem as the other Girl Scout in the way I thought the poet had intended. I won the poetry contest. The prize included six months of theatrical training—on Saturdays. Who knows? Maybe I could have been an actress. But Mami said, "No." Such was not to be because those hated Saturdays were enema days—not theatrical training days.

A big difference between my friends and me growing up was that my mother was the teacher at the schools I attended; when I was in high school, she became the principal. She started as what was called a "normalist teacher," as she had just two years of university education. Later, she earned her bachelor's and master's degrees—both in education. She was originally a mathematics teacher, and she was the teacher at the elementary school when I was young.

Elementary schools at that time didn't have kindergartens—they started with first grade. Each class had the same teacher for three years. So if you were lucky, you had two good teachers for your six years of elementary school.

When I was five, Mami brought me with her to the elementary school where she was teaching. This was both to keep me busy—and out of trouble—and to help her feel more secure by knowing my whereabouts. She placed me with the first-grade class. Her instructions to me were along the lines of "Sit there and don't make trouble." When it was time for me to go to first grade, I think that the teacher told my mother that I had learned everything I was going to learn in first grade, so they put me in second grade. And Mami had just taken me there to be babysat.

Having a teacher for three years might be good except if the teacher didn't like you—then you were doomed. My brother, Tomas, had a teacher he didn't like for three years. The teacher I had for both second and third grade was an old lady who I realized later didn't like my aunts because they were good looking and young and were dating GIs from the naval base five miles away. I think she resented their youth and liberty. Fair or not, I paid the price. When that teacher asked me to read in front of the class one time too many, she pushed me aside and chastised me for reading from memory and not from the book. I thought you had to be somewhat dumb not to repeat seven hundred times "Peter throw the ball—throw the ball, Peter" and not know it by heart. She never even explained what "reading from memory" meant; she just took my books away. So throughout the rest of the year, I learned to read from newspapers rather than reading my schoolbooks. That teacher never had me read in front of the class again.

In third grade, I was transferred to a different group without the old teacher. I never knew if it meant I was dumber than the other students in her class or if she was just tired of my presence. I never found out, but it damaged my self-esteem early in my life. In fourth grade, I had to go to another school because Mami and my stepfather moved. That teacher was very, very good. In fact, the school is now named for her. When she gave me my first test, I got an "E" for "excellent." I remember that vividly. I went to her and told her that I didn't think my paper had been graded correctly. She asked me why, and I told her that I wasn't an E student, that I was an S, S+ (S was for satisfactory). I had gotten low self-esteem from my second- and third-grade teacher who had always graded me with S. Perhaps this new teacher had discovered that I was better than the previous one had thought. This was the first time in my life where I believed I might be better than I had been told to believe. She said I was an E student. From that moment, I became motivated to always be an E student.

We moved again, so I started fifth grade at a new school in Fajardo. Mami was always looking for the best teacher in whatever school I was in to make sure I was put in the best class. She never sent me to Catholic school; she always sent me to public school because (according to her) the teachers at the Catholic schools were the ones that could not survive the rigors of public schools and their types of students.

My year of fifth grade was interrupted, however, when I was sent to New York City for three months. My aunt lived in New York City, and I was sent so that she could take me to Belleview Hospital to see if they had a treatment for my congenital megacolon. I remember being in the hospital and being in front of a group of people all dressed in white, which I now believe to have been a grand rounds. For whatever reason, I received no treatment and came back to Puerto Rico, reconnecting with my fifth-grade class. Sixth grade was fine except for the principal. She was cruel and would hit you if you misbehaved; she seemed especially to target the boys. I had no problems—if she would have hit me, Mami would have taken care of her.

When I got a B on one of my English tests in seventh grade, I went crying to Mami: "I have failed. My life is finished." And Mami said it was a test, not a grade. So I became myself again. But that grade ruined my straight E (A equivalent) average and was a blow to my self-esteem since I had vowed to be an E student always.

At that time, I was very actively fist fighting as well. I was the defender of women and if anyone said something or did something wrong to a friend of mine, I had a fistfight. I think I got that strength of conviction from my mother. It is amazing that I survived all of that without any broken bones.

I survived high school; Mami had made sure that I had the best teacher in every single class again. We were a small group—no more than thirty. We all knew each other, including everybody's idiosyncrasies. There was always a teacher's pet. In our case, it was a boy from the next town. I really liked him, but instead of showing him that I liked him, I competed with him. I would get an A and he would get an A. It was neck and neck. All the time. He was very brilliant. Being brilliant isn't enough by itself, though. You have to use that brilliance.

When Mami became the principal of the junior high school I had attended, I felt that all eyes were on me. I had to be the best.

I simply couldn't fail. There was never any room to be weak. Not all my teachers appreciated that my mother was the principal, and some of my friends didn't, either. I remember coming down the staircase to meet my friends, and hearing them say, "I bet you that Mrs. Flores [Mami] got her an A in Spanish." I did get an A, but not because of Mami—I studied a lot for that A.

In my last year of high school, I took trigonometry not because I needed the credit to graduate but to be with my friends. That teacher was very jealous of my mother. She called me to the front of the class and said, "Tell your mother that I gave you your first B." With a B in trigonometry, my average dropped from a 4.0 to a 3.98. I was still the top student in my class and class valedictorian, but my grades were affected by the jealousy between this teacher and my mother. I still don't understand why the trigonometry teacher did that. This was another one of those times when I felt betrayed by a teacher.

I took the test for entering the University of Puerto Rico when I was a junior because Mami said, "You only have Spanish 101 to finish. And you are going to college in August." And I said, "Mami, if you make me take the test and send me to college without my friends, then I will fail." She replied, "You are going to take the test now. And in case you fail, you'll take it again next year, but you're just not going to kind of linger around here all because of only one class." Mami was strong. They say in Africa that when elephants walk, they kill ants. My mother was part elephant. She would destroy anything in her path that was not doing what she thought was best. So I took the test, and by the grace of God I got the highest grade of anyone taking the test that year, including all the seniors. I stayed at the high school for my senior year, and when it was time to take the test again, I was there just eating ice cream, looking around the classroom at all the students killing themselves to finish. The principal of the high school never told anyone of my grade on the test, so I blended in my senior year and graduated with honors at age sixteen in 1961.

In my hometown, you could send a letter to the mayor, to the pharmacist, to the superintendent, and to the principal (that was my mother) with just their names. Mami trained a whole generation, and sometimes even today I find people who say, "I am who I am because of your mother." For a while, she taught seventh grade. I asked her why she wasn't teaching high school, and she said that she wanted students when they were still children, just getting ready to move into adolescence, so that she still could mold their brains. But she wasn't always completely sensitive. For example, she had this ruler that was called "Catalina." The whole school knew about that ruler. Before you could enter her room, you had to recite all the multiplication tables. (To this day, I know them by heart; I don't have to use the calculator unless there are big numbers involved.) And if you did not know them because you were sloppy or didn't want to study, you got a little Catalina on your leg. We framed the ruler for Mami and gave it to her when she retired. In her later years, Mami and I used to laugh when she said, "I probably would be in prison now if I used Catalina with the students today." The biggest school in my hometown is now named after my mother.

In addition to being the mathematics teacher, she also taught science, and she could go to the blackboard and do a perfect circle with one piece of chalk. Mami could talk about mathematics in such a beautiful way.

She always wore a flower on her dress because her name was Flores, which means "flower" in Spanish. All my adult life I have worn a broach, and when asked why, I say that Mami always wore a flower, and I wear the broach in honor of my mother.

She did something else that wouldn't be acceptable today. Her classroom was divided into rows—A, B, C, D, F. And depending on how you behaved and by your grade, she would sit you in the corresponding row. One day, she gave a quiz, and I got maybe a C. She sat me in the F row for a week. I have never been so embarrassed. Maybe that's why I studied so hard for the rest of my life. I decided I was never going to sit anywhere but in the A row. She treated everyone the same. If my achievements were not up to par, then I had to bear the consequences of my actions in her class. She had expectations of me, and I worked so hard not to fail her.

Every four years, I would see someone coming to the house in Fajardo trying to get Mami to run for mayor. She would always say no. She was more interested in making sure that each generation got educated while they were in school and ready to be productive adults. And there were many times that she was asked to be superintendent of schools in my hometown. She would always laugh so hard and say, "No, are you out of your mind? You think for some lousy dollars I am going to take all the responsibility of telling everybody what to do and no one will obey me? My classroom is my kingdom. And no one tells me what to do."

From my sophomore year through half of my senior year, Mami served as principal of a high school in a town an hour and a half away. Mami did not drive, so she was driven to the school. She would leave Monday morning, return Tuesday evening, leave again Wednesday morning, and return Friday evening. At the same time, she was studying for her master's in education. My brother, Tomas, and I were at home with our stepfather and the lady who used to make meals and clean the house. The rules were not changed, however, just because she was not there. The expectations continued. Studying was obligatory. Tomas and I still had household duties to perform. No matter where I was—at the library or chit-chatting with my friends—my curfew was at nine o'clock at night, and wherever I was I had better speed it up to get home. The church bells were my clock—last ding, and I had better be in front of the door, or else.

As far as I was concerned, my mother always preferred Tomas to me. I was the girl who always got the good grades and did all the things that were expected of me. My brother could always be pardoned for everything because Mami was so enamored with him. If there was reprimanding or scolding or even hitting, I always got it double because as mother would say—"You are the oldest." And I think some of it was also that I looked like my father.

Throughout our lives, my brother and I were on good terms—but he had some sort of jealousy over me being in medicine. He always felt that I got more than he did, while I kept thinking that he was the one without complications. He was handsome, intelligent, and had no constipation. His life felt uncomplicated as far as I was concerned. He got the bicycle, the piano, the larger car, the horse. From my perspective, he had it all.

* * *

When I was in high school, I was part of a group of five girls. We were friends for life, and we called ourselves the "Five Signorinas." But even though we were friends, we were also very competitive with each other. I think they thought my belonging to the group was a good thing because my mother was the principal of a school. But I was smart and worked hard to succeed because I wanted to. As a group, we belonged to all the clubs and were active in every extracurricular activity. I was the funny one of the group. I laughed at myself because of my intestinal problems. I took to heart the words of Juan de Dios Peza in his poem "Reir Ilorando" ("To Laugh While Crying")—"Nobody trust the merriment of laughter, because in those beings devoured by pain, the soul groans when the face laughs!"

I challenged anybody. I challenged myself more than I was challenged by them. I also felt that I was the underdog—my mother was the principal. One girl's father was a doctor. One girl's parents were wealthy. So I saw the gradient and I played the game. In our town, there were divisions of classes and jobs and people and who's who. I often won, but I did it without threatening them.

There was a program on television with school competitions. We would go to the government channel, which was where the competition was held, and we would compete in every category—even the ones we didn't know. I remember memorizing the names of all the dogs in the world so that when they would show me a picture, I would know which breed it was. We were competing against the most important and intelligent groups of girls' and boys' schools in the capital. Although we were from eastern Puerto Rico, we came in second to them. For me, that was very important because they were from the best schools.

We were all very close in our high school years—very close, but very competitive, even helping to clean the trigonometry teacher's house on Saturdays. Go figure. We were the good kids in the school. Every teacher loved us and wanted us in their class.

During high school, Mami used to give me 25 cents to buy myself a snack from the food cart in front of the school. When I was either thirteen or fourteen, I thought I should get myself a bra. So I saved that money and went to the Bella Hess store and put a bra the size I thought I was—30AA—on layaway. I paid religiously. But my body grew faster than my layaway balance. By the time I was able to get my layaway bra, I had outgrown both the band and the cup size. I was debating whether to even try it on. I did, but it did not fit at all. Basically, I could not breathe. My next bra was a 34 B—one year later. As I reached maturity, my cup size changed again but not much. I learned, however, the larger size bras are much more expensive than the 30AA bra.

Every summer for ten days, every town in Puerto Rico honors its patron saint. When I was fifteen years old, I was proclaimed the Queen of the Plaza during the patron saint days in Fajardo. It was fun, but it was a lot of hoopla and money for such a short period of time.

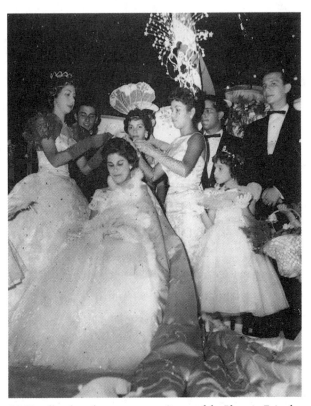

Dr. Novello when she was a young Queen of the Plaza in Fajardo, Puerto Rico.

When I was an adult, maybe in 1976, all the previous town queens were invited to go down the main street wearing a beautiful gown and crown to re-create the time when they had been named Queen of the Plaza. My husband was in Washington, D.C., and Tomas, my brother, refused to go with me and act like my date, so I walked the whole distance alone. I was wearing a beautiful velvet dress adorned all over with beads. My hair had looked fine until the shower faucet got half of it wet. I wore the crown quite intentionally placed so that no one could detect the hair mishap.

All the former queens had gathered in the plaza of my home-town. In honor of International Women's Day, one former queen was to be selected by the emcee pulling a name out of a glass jar. The emcee was a friend of my mother's and a friend of mine, and lo and behold—he pulled my name out of the jar. I was not pleased as I thought people were thinking it was an arranged win. I was not about to let that happen. I requested that all the names that were left in the glass jar be read out loud. My mother was about to faint. But the names were read, and by sheer luck I had really won.

I was proud and my mother was relieved. You never knew what that emcee might have done to get my mother's approval. This time, he was not dishonest in any way. I was proud to give myself the place of honor that day.

Because I had completed first grade so early, I was just sixteen when I graduated from high school, turning seventeen when I started college at the University of Puerto Rico at Rio Piedras. I decided to major in natural sciences. That meant I would take biology and chemistry and so forth. My friends were majoring in social and political sciences and home economics, which meant I was the only one in natural sciences from my class. And I was still dealing with my congenital megacolon.

CHAPTER 2

A Kindly Professor and the Mayo Clinic Saved My Life

When I was about to enter my sophomore year in college and Tomas was newly enrolled in his first year of college, Mami decided to take us to the town where she had lived with my father. She said she was afraid that Tomas would marry one of his half sisters unknowingly. We had heard that my father had married the maid and sired about eight children before his death, Martin being the oldest.

Mother, Tomas, and I were dressed to kill. We were going back to where our mother had been rejected by our father—and where a maid was made to feel more important than the mother of his oldest children.

We entered the house, and I remember it being very large with a huge circular balcony; high columns held up the top floor. There were many children running, screaming, and jumping. We were met by a woman, somewhat chubby, average looks, big belly, and, as I recall, lacking two front teeth: our former maid, Canda. And there was my mother—perfectly dressed and poised, almost twenty years later. Mami proceeded to do the introductions. I was the spitting image of my father, while my brother Tomas had my mother's face but almost the exact body type of my father. I don't think that Canda was ready for these two children who came back to remind her of what had happened almost twenty years ago.

My mother then asked me to kiss Canda and give her a hug. I was incredulous that Mami was making this request of me. *What?* Of course, I said no. Mami proceeded to ask me again, this time more forcefully, to which I said, "I see no reason to do this, but if you have an explanation that is acceptable to me, perhaps I will." Mami looked at me and said, "You are going to kiss and hug this woman and thank her, because if this woman did not exist perhaps today you would be one of those children jumping all around this house and would not be where you are today—in college and graduating in two years."

I understood vividly what she said, and I kissed the woman. If Mother could forgive—who was I to act bigger in my persona than she? We stayed overnight and left the next morning, having learned a lesson of humility and forgiveness of an absent father whose children never had our opportunities.

A few months later, Tomas and I each got a check for $5,000 for what seemed to be an inheritance from our father. Canda had sold the house and the farm we had visited and left the island with all of her children in tow. To this day, I do not know what happened to her or my half brothers and half sisters.

Later, when I was Surgeon General, I went back in uniform to visit Puerto Rico and vaccinate the children in Jayuya—my father's hometown. My aunts from my father's side took a picture of me in uniform next to a picture of my father in his policeman's uniform. Today, that picture hangs in all its splendor in the surviving aunts' living room.

* * *

I was eighteen years old and a sophomore in college when my mother and I were approached by a new neighbor who asked me when I was due to give birth. She noted my enlarged abdomen and assumed I was pregnant. I was mortified. College had been different from growing up in a small town where everyone knew the circumstances of my condition. But in college, everything changed—the perception, the looks, the subtle gossip. I was annoyed, but I had lived with it all my life. Why did it have to change? And if I had been assumed to be pregnant, then a flat belly connoted that I had had an abortion. Even more mortifying!

But now, my mother and I both went into explanation mode. While Mami was still in the discussion, I went into the bathroom and drank twelve ounces of castor oil. That is all I remember until about twenty-four hours later when I emerged out of a semiconscious state of emptying my bowel. I begged my mother to put an end to this part of my life. To me, it didn't matter who or when, but I needed an operation now!

Mami did find a doctor who was willing to do the surgery. I needed to end what I now characterized as a continual agonizing embarrassment. Unfortunately for me, the doctor she found was a cardiac surgeon at the Teacher's Hospital where my mother carried her health insurance. He was short and cocky and performed my gastrointestinal operation without the appropriate knowledge. He removed thirty-two inches of my large intestine that lacked the Auerbach nervous plexus, and he then stitched the residual intestine to the inner anal sphincter. This created another problem as it hampered the anal spinchter's ability to open and close as expected with normal bowel movements.

Although his intentions were presumably good, the results were worse than the constipation I had endured for eighteen years. At the end of the surgery, he had created a recto-vaginal fistula (an abnormal connection), which over the next three years would produce constant leakage for which I had to use large quantities of period pads, and, at times, diapers. He also created a rectal stricture when he stitched my colon to the anal sphincter rather than performing a short-term colostomy. I now began to get my first glimpse of hell.

When I came out of that surgery, I was not in very good shape. I stayed in the Teacher's Hospital recovering for three to four weeks. I remember the drains coming out of the right side of my lower abdomen. When I left the hospital, I went to stay at Mami Loli's house. During that stay, my operation wound burst open so the incision had to be cleaned thoroughly; my aunt did it all. Still, I had to go back to the hospital. The opened incision finally closed through secondary healing. My wound had to be cleaned every single day, and I didn't heal well. The mesh that had been inserted in my right side was finally pulled out; at the time of my surgery, a mesh was left in place to allow drainage inside to come out. My aunt gave me antibiotics and while taking care of me reinforced my idea about studying medicine to help others.

And since I had no other information or knowledge, I was also always afraid that I had lost my virginity because of the fistula. I never told my mother anything about this worry. Maybe I shouldn't have hidden it from her. But there were many things that I did hide from Mami. There were so many things that I wanted and needed to know, but I just couldn't burden her.

And although I did not discover it until about ten years later when I tried to get pregnant, the doctor had cut one of my Fallopian tubes. In addition, the mesh that was on the right side caused an infection that damaged the second Fallopian tube. I was now sterile for life at age eighteen. And he never said a word.

I had recovered adequately enough from the surgery and its complications to start my junior year in college. But I was still competitive and I took twenty-one credits. I didn't care that I had just had surgery in June. August was the month when classes started, and I wanted to be there. There wasn't a single easy class. I was not going to be left behind because of my surgery; in my mind that would have been a failure. I challenged myself. I wore diapers for six months, going through that first semester of my junior year in college. This was a significant hit to my self-esteem. In your late teenage years when you're supposed to be good looking and attractive to the opposite sex, I was not. Instead I was wearing diapers. So I didn't date—I just studied. If anyone would have discovered that I was wearing diapers, I would have died of embarrassment. So I pretended like nothing unusual was happening in my life and carried on normally. I did not dwell on the negative—I always found a way to be positive. I didn't let anything stop me. My body was broken—but not my brain. Once again laughing while crying kept me going.

I cannot tell you if being called pregnant at eighteen was worse than having a constant, uncontrolled amount of liquid stool coming out of your vagina, even as you washed yourself constantly. The embarrassment and the smell were accompanied by intense pain in my lower back. I learned then what it is to smile despite the pain. I also learned to go into bathrooms first when they were empty and to wait to leave last when they were not full so that no one would know that the smell was coming from me.

As luck would have it, every Saturday morning I had to go to the Teacher's Hospital to see the doctor who had done my surgery for a rectal dilatation. This was to open the obstruction that was made in my rectum by the "pull-through" maneuver that stitched my colon to my rectal sphincter. For the dilatation procedure, I had to have anesthesia.

Every Friday afternoon during my college years, I took "publico" transportation to get to my hometown of Fajardo—more than an hour-long trip, and longer, depending on traffic. During my freshman and sophomore years, I had gone home for my Saturday enemas and to study. As a junior and senior, I came home for my rectal dilatations at the Teacher's Hospital and to study.

I took a Spanish class during college on Friday afternoons. Although the teacher used to show my tests to the class as an example of how to write essays when taking a test, apparently she wasn't always pleased by my attendance.

I always felt very good about having studied so hard because in the long run, it pays. However, I knew that this teacher was not very happy when I took a Friday off to get home earlier so that I could then spend all day Saturday having my rectal dilatations resulting in only one lost day. I didn't know how seriously this affected her until my grades came. I truly felt that because all my tests were being shown to the class—as perfect—my grade was going to be an A. To my dismay, my grade was a B. I was shocked, not only because I had studied so hard for the final test and knew that I had aced it but also because with that B I was unable to graduate from college with a cum laude. She will never know how her actions affected me, and I will never forget what she did. If I ever knew her name, I have now buried it.

I cannot remember the name of my college biology teacher either, but she was one of my heroes. She always felt that I could be somebody and challenged me to move out of my comfort zone. I used her as an example when I wrote my entrance letter for my medical school application. I don't think she ever knew. But I will always remember her for helping me become a doctor.

I had wanted to be a doctor since I was a little girl. But I didn't tell my friends, and I especially didn't tell Mami. At home, everybody was a teacher or a nurse, and Mami was the principal of the school. I was afraid she was going to say, "And what happened to teaching? Are you embarrassed about what we do?" I was afraid of the rejection and laughter and scorn from my peers, so I never said anything about becoming a doctor. I also didn't tell my mother because I didn't think the financial burden of medical school was a reasonable thing to ask of someone who earned a teacher's salary. I didn't want to add to her economic worries.

I went to take my MCATs and applied for medical school without telling her. When I entered the room for the MCAT, my fellow test takers had many books open and were reading and studying. It was the first time I realized that there was such a thing as a Kaplan book with which you could review your knowledge before medical school. I knew nothing of such a book or such reviews. I just went and took my test. If I would have had mentors in my life, I probably would have benefited significantly. However, I must have done well on my test as I was called for an interview at the medical school.

I went to my mother the day I got the letter that said I had an interview for medical school. "Mami, tomorrow I have an interview for going to medical school." I told her, "You know I have always been in hospitals—all the summers until I was eighteen. It is something I want to do." And I remember she said without hesitation, "As long as there is a bank that gives me a loan for your tuition, you're going to medical school." I never expected that kind of reaction.

It seemed that everybody who wanted to go to medical school prepared by visiting the "referral" doctor whose recommendation made it possible to enter. Mine was an imposing, powerful woman with a skeleton in full view in her office. I think her name was Dr. Dexter. Her reputation was such that I knew she was very fond of physicians' children—the ones who were enrolled in premed. This course of study at the university almost always assured entrance to medical school. I had had nothing like that. Mami wanted me to have a bachelor's degree in hand. This was in case anything failed along the way—I would have the means to earn a living. Once I had that bachelor's degree, I would then be able to apply to medical school. So when Dr. Dexter and I met, she told me that I had small hands that would be very good for dentistry. At that moment, I decided to bypass her advice and proceeded to do everything required for entrance to medical school on my own.

The interview itself was very strange. The medical school professors and I were all seated around a circular table. The most senior professors asked me a couple of questions. To my right was the psychiatrist making little doodles as I spoke. They really were trying to intimidate me. In the end, they accepted only five women out of the total class of fifty. They even said to me, "You're a woman, you will be taking the position of a man. How do you feel about that?" And I answered that I loved medicine. All my life I had been in hospitals. I knew exactly what I wanted to do to help people. Then they asked me, "What if we don't accept you?" And I said, "Then I will apply to be a medical technologist and will reapply to medical school next year."

When the list of students who were accepted to medical school at the University of Puerto Rico School of Medicine at San Juan was posted, I was not on the list—at least I thought I wasn't. I asked for the alternate list—the ones waitlisted in case somebody dropped out of the class. I wasn't there either. My name has always created problems for me because "Antonia" often gets confused with "Antonio." I was devastated. Then I asked to look at the alphabetic list of those who were going to medical school. I was there! But with the name of Antonio, not Antonia. They had put down the wrong name. I got into medical school. I didn't have to be a medical technologist for a year and then reapply.

Mami gave me the wings to be whatever I wanted to be. It was such a good feeling—such trust in me. She made sure I had a place to live, money for gas, and a car so that I no longer had to take "publico" transportation. She knew that I would be studying every night at somebody else's home. That car was a red sports car. So now I was not only a medical student, I was also a hot-rodder in a beautiful red convertible car. All she expected of me was to pass and do well.

My very best friend was Nora, who was about five years my junior. (She is still alive, recovering from bilateral breast cancer.) I met Nora when she was in college, and I was in my first year of medical school. We got introduced through her sister, who was one of my high school friends. I was always welcome in her home when I couldn't bear to be anywhere else. Her mother and her father never protested about the smell. She and I learned to laugh about it and did everything together. She never put a napkin on her nose. To her I had no smell. On her face I never saw a grimace, disdain, or a frown.

I was "Toña," her friend for life. We have always been the closest that any friends can be because we survived—we survived that time in my life. I am so thankful for Nora because I believe you have to have a friend you trust and believe for life. She never laughed at my weirdest dreams nor rejected me for my acquired problems. She was my shoulder to cry on; my secrets were safe with her.

* * *

During the time of my recto-vaginal fistula, one of my aunts came to the house. When she walked in, she said, "Oh, my God, what a stink." My stepfather slapped her. He said, "In this house, if you're not going to have empathy, you are not welcome. She has enough to bear for you to be her aunt and criticize what she cannot control." That day my stepfather became a giant in front of my eyes.

I was thrown out of two boarding houses during my first year of medical school. These situations pushed me down even more into depression and low self-esteem. And I learned how little tolerance people have for the ones who have no one to protect and speak for them.

The woman who ran the first boarding house said that I had to leave because there was always a little too much grain on the shower floor after I had finished bathing. She told me that she couldn't take a shower after I had gotten out because there was so much dung on the floor. The grain of stool, I guess. She made me feel like dirt. I knew that I would take a shower and when I dried myself off, the towel was already dirty. So it must have been a huge fistula.

I didn't want to tell Mami that I had to move because, knowing my mother, she would have come and given the lady a little bit of her mind. I went to the house of one of my medical school colleagues instead. His mother eventually said I had to leave because people were saying that here is her son and there is a woman in the same room. God forgive me, but I think he was probably gay! However, I think the real reason that she asked me to leave was my smell that came from the mixing of stool and vaginal fluids and the amount of the drainage. It hurt terribly. This medical school colleague would even buy me the large period pad box every other day and bring it into the house. Upon my return to Puerto Rico after my surgery at the Mayo Clinic when I was twenty-two, I saw the mother of my medical school classmate at a gathering I attended. I gave her the biggest hug, and I said to her in her ear, "Tell me if I smell now." And she started crying.

I had a crush on a boy when I was in college. I knew that he had a girlfriend already. Every time I would pass the girlfriend, she would be with a clump of girls who looked rich and whose parents were rich as well. She would snicker or say something under her breath as I passed by. And then I went to medical school, and lo and behold, who was seated two seats from me? There he was; we were seated alphabetically. Years later, when I was at the National Institutes of Health (NIH), I was responsible for hosting a research week at the University of Puerto Rico Medical School and I invited every director of each NIH Institute to lecture regarding the latest research pertinent to that field of expertise. And who was sitting in the first row? Yes, him. It must have been a shock to him that the person who was bringing research to the University of Puerto Rico was the same one whom his former girlfriend, now wife, was always belittling. It brings up a life lesson—never disregard anyone on your way to the top because you never know where you are going to find them.

> "Never disregard anyone on your way to the top because you never know where you are going to find them."

We had a very sad experience during my first semester of medical school. A very beautiful woman who was in the class ahead of us took her own life. She gave herself an injection of potassium chloride while lying in bed with a stethoscope on her chest. We found out when the anatomy teacher, who I think had a slight crush on her, came to class crying. That was when we knew that not everyone survives medical school.

During the second semester of my first year of medical school, the recto-vaginal fistula was getting worse. The secretions were uncontrollable, and I needed a whole box of period pads daily to feel at least somewhat clean. My medical school colleagues who sat near me used to move a little bit farther away as we listened to lectures. I would get to school in the afternoons and plug in my microscope and my heating pad. The heating pad was for the lower back pain that was so intense from the fistula.

With Easter break approaching that spring, my medical school physiology teacher recommended that I have a colostomy. I asked her why and how long I would have it. She said maybe forever. At twenty-one years old that felt like a death sentence. She suggested that I discuss it with my mother, which I did. I told Mami that I would kill myself if she agreed. She said it was my body and my decision. By now, it was almost three years since the surgery that was supposed to have been the "cure" had occurred.

The physiology professor further recommended that I make an appointment with the Chief of Surgery at the medical school to learn more about the colostomy. She said, "You go see him. You get a colostomy over the week of Easter and then come back and take your finals." I really wanted to be clean—I felt I didn't belong because of the smell. So I did make an appointment, but when I saw the doctor, for some reason—call it intuition—I said I didn't want to be examined because I was menstruating. I don't know why I lied. But he did not examine me. This made my physiology teacher angry with me.

When I went in for my next Saturday's rectal dilatation for the rectal stricture, the cardiac surgeon refused to see me because I had visited another doctor for consultation. In addition, although I did not know it, the Chief of Surgery whom I had seen—but who had not examined me—was the archenemy of the cardiac surgeon who had performed my congenital megacolon surgery. The Chief of Surgery had refused to allow the cardiac surgeon to become a member of the American College of Surgeons. I paid the price of that infighting.

So there I was at age twenty-one with no doctor, a recto-vaginal fistula, chronic cystitis, a rectal stricture, and no explanation whatsoever of why he dropped me. I felt lonely and dejected. No referrals nor follow-up appointments. Sick and depressed and nowhere

"I promised myself that I was never going to treat any patient of mine that way or have any patient of mine feel that way."

to go. I fell through the cracks of the health-care system. In my own personal hell. Rejected and with no self-esteem. I left in a daze. The doctors had failed me—and, at the time, doctors were viewed as gods. I never told my mother anything about this. I always had believed that Mami felt a sense of guilt about my condition while Tomas was so healthy. I did not want to add to her burden—although this was never spoken between us. I was not going to add to her problems.

From that moment on, I became very empathetic toward people in my type of situation. Poor people who, unlike their rich friends, have no way to get an appointment. Poor people who are basically stuck with the same doctor because they think there are no options, or because they don't know where else to go. I promised myself that I was never going to treat any patient of mine that way or have any patient of mine feel that way.

I had missed several of my Monday morning physiology laboratories during my second semester of medical school due to the rectal dilatations I received on Saturdays. I received no pain medications after the procedure, and the pain I experienced on Sunday and Monday often precluded my driving back to school in time for my morning physiology labs. My car had a stick shift, and the pain was just too overwhelming when I pressed the clutch.

My physiology professor, the one who had recommended the colostomy, came to me and said, "Don't you worry. I will help you repeat these physiology laboratories." And I said, "Okay." When my grades came, I had an E in physiology, which meant that I needed to remove the deficiency. To do so, I needed to complete the laboratories that I had missed. I visited my professor at the beginning of the summer to take the laboratories as she had requested. Instead, she said, "Oh, darling, I'm so sorry, but I'm writing a grant for the National Institutes of Health, and I won't be able to help you." She gave no further explanations, nor did she show empathy or provide alternatives. She must have seen the look of pain and horror on my face because she suggested that losing a year of medical school was no big deal. She said that she had lost one and look where she was now—my professor.

I thought my world was crumbling again. What would I do? I had no hope or future options. It was June. What would I tell my mother? She was paying all this money for me to go to medical school, and now I was going to have to tell her that I flunked out because my teacher would not help me complete the laboratories I had missed— despite having promised that I could complete them and that she would help me. The picture was overwhelming. The doors were closing on me. All the sacrifices my mother had made for me and all her efforts on my behalf might come to naught. I was sobbing as I came down the stairs at the medical school. I was devastated. If ever I felt like ending everything, that was the moment.

On my way down the stairs, I ran into the American doctor who was my professor of histology, Dr. Josel Szepsenwol (Chepi, as we called him), and he asked me what was wrong. I said that I had just seen my physiology teacher. In between sobs, I told him that she had previously told me she was going to repeat my labs so that I could remove the E, and now she was telling me that she had to write a grant and thus could not help me. He said, "I told that witch to give you a D and let you pass. And she said no because you have a B equivalent, and she wasn't going to make it easier and that you would have to repeat the labs."

He took my hand, and then he said, "Have you ever heard of the Mayo Clinic?" Me? A kid from the little town of Fajardo, Puerto Rico? I said, "No, I don't know anything about it." He said, "I'm referring you there. I'm going to call them, and I'm going to make you an appointment." And he did—he got me an appointment in October, which meant I would miss the first semester of my second year of medical school. At the same time, Mami Loli, my favorite aunt, had developed renal failure accompanied by severe high blood pressure and had to start dialysis at Bethesda Naval Hospital (now Walter Reed) in Maryland. Bethesda was the only place that was doing dialysis in those very early days of kidney treatment, and Mami Loli was married to a man who had served in the Navy. My mother paid for my trip to the Mayo Clinic in Rochester, Minnesota, as well as accommodations in the area, while she accompanied Mami Loli to Bethesda. Because I was a medical student, I did get my care at the Mayo Clinic at a significant discount from the usual cost. In addition, as a medical student, I could pay off the remainder of my debt as I was able. That is what we did. Otherwise, I knew it would not work as well, especially if Mami had to worry about paying another bill.

* * *

The little girl from Puerto Rico arrived in Rochester, Minnesota, in October. I had never experienced cold weather before, so I was dressed like a Puerto Rican with a jacket. Because I had been the Queen of the USO in Fajardo, I attended USO events at the naval base in Puerto Rico. At one of the USO events were some Navy personnel from Minnesota who were stationed at the base. When I said I had to go to the Mayo Clinic, one of these men from Minnesota said he thought his parents would be very pleased to have me as their guest. And they were. They picked me up at the airport. They took me to their house in Dawson, Minnesota. I slept in their house, and they took me to all my first appointments. They did everything that could be done—and all for a complete stranger. Mami sent them presents—all the other children in the family were girls. They were such good people with good hearts. I will always remember them with much affection.

My first doctor's appointment at the Mayo Clinic was with surgical proctologist Dr. Markham Anderson. To me he looked like the television doctor, Marcus Welby, MD, from the 1960s and '70s, and he acted the same. He was kind. He listened. He treated me with the utmost respect even though I was only a medical student. He helped me tremendously to overcome the fear of the consultation, the unknown, and the loneliness. He examined me with a specific focus on the rectal stricture and ordered a colonoscopy. His nurse was Pearl, and, like Dr. Anderson, she was very sensitive. She, in my eyes, looked and acted like Florence Nightingale.

The Mayo Clinic strove to treat all patients humanely and respectfully. Everyone on your floor had the same symptoms and maybe required the same tests. So the day I had my colonoscopy, so did everyone else. We had all taken our enemas, we had all spent the entire night in the bathroom because of the laxatives we had to take beforehand, and we were all walking the same way. We didn't have to hide that we were in agony, and we all answered the same questions for the lady in front. That gave us real empathy for those around us. We felt safe.

Dr. Anderson then decided that my next consultation would be with a gynecologist for the recto-vaginal fistula. That doctor seemed capable but distant compared to Dr. Anderson. He proceeded to examine me and looked slightly puzzled. He said, "What is the reason you are here?" I explained everything again—the stricture, the fistula, and so forth—and he proceeded to tell me that he found no fistula whatsoever. In addition, he suggested I should go see a psychologist (meaning that he thought I could be crazy, even malingering, and making all of this up). I was in shock. The Mayo Clinic thinks I am malingering my symptoms? I was now lonely and feeling even more desperate. But I knew I had real physical problems, and I wanted to prove him wrong before he called a psych consultant.

I left and went to see Dr. Anderson. He was kind and listened to me as he saw me in tears. He read the report from the gynecologist. He never gave up on me. He decided to do a fistulogram to document the presence of the fistula. To our amazement, the fistulogram, which uses an X-ray and dye, not only demonstrated the presence of the fistula but also the presence of a not uncommon complication found whenever there is a genetic malformation to begin with: I had two vaginas and two uteri. The gynecologist who had seen me found that the septum separating the two vaginas was intact but was not able to detect the connection between one of the vaginas and the rectum. Without the fistulogram and Dr. Anderson's persistence, I would have been mislabeled and once again kept in the dark. I was not crazy or malingering after all. A fistula was present as it had been since my congenital megacolon surgery three years before.

Dr. Anderson scheduled the surgery to fix the fistula and associated issues. The day before my surgery, this very cocky female anesthesiologist came in and was very patronizing to me because I was a medical student. She said, "I am going to give you a spinal tap." And I said, "You know, I would really appreciate it if you would put me to sleep. I am afraid. I am out of my country and my comfort zone. I don't have anybody with me." And she looked at me with disdain.

Next thing I knew I was at the surgery. I was on the table, and she gave me the spinal. And then she turned me face down so that Dr. Anderson could come in and do the surgery. Because he was such a kind and humane doctor, he came in and tickled my nose.

My face was looking down and my rear was up. He asked me how I was doing. The spinal had taken effect, and I was not breathing. I guess my eyes must have been out of their sockets. He turned me over immediately and started giving me oxygen. I was looking at the anesthesiologist, who was pacing back and forth pulling her hair out. I had told her not to give me a spinal tap. Finally, she left, and Dr. Anderson said, "We are going to put you to sleep. We are not missing this opportunity."

Dr. Anderson operated on me, fixing my stricture, retaining one healthy vagina, closing the fistula and removing the second vagina. He tended to me as a father. He came to see me every single day in my room to check whether I had passed stools. And I was embarrassed beyond belief, but on the first day that I had, he was there to watch. He had constructed the missing pieces and fixed the messes that were created during my surgery in Puerto Rico. He wanted to verify that what he had done was workable. I never imagined that someone in his specialty, in charge of the whole department, would come and watch me going to the bathroom to see if everything was correct.

The Mayo Clinic changed my life. I always felt badly that I was never able to tell Dr. Anderson or Pearl that I had become Surgeon General, because they died before that happened. Dr. Anderson's kindness extended to me personally. While I was still in Minnesota and he knew I needed money, he would always find a way for me to babysit. In addition, he and Pearl would take me to dinner. I always felt very appreciative of both of them. And they each hold a very special place in my heart. God knows what my life would have been like without Dr. Anderson ordering a fistulogram.

I didn't need to stay in the hospital during my entire recovery, but I did need to be close by and come into the hospital for periodic visits until the discharge was finalized. I had developed a friendship with one of my hospital roommates—a women recovering from varicose vein surgery. She invited me to stay at her home where I continued my recovery and babysat her five children. Later, I stayed a few days with the young woman who rented the television sets to the Mayo Clinic. After three months at the Mayo Clinic, when I had made a full recovery, I returned to Puerto Rico. That was in December.

When I flew home, my mother was on another plane that day, accompanying my aunt's body home. Mami Loli had died while she was at Bethesda. I saw my mother so thin and so frail while my grandmother was crying for my aunt. I felt very sad when I saw my mother bringing my dead aunt home. No one paid attention to her sacrifice—they only cried for my dead aunt. Much was expected of my mother as the eldest; very little of her stepsisters. Seeing all their pain and knowing that my aunt had died of kidney disease was the moment that I decided to become a nephrologist. This way, I knew that if anyone else in my family got sick, they would be properly informed about their disease and offered choices.

* * *

Through the kindness of strangers and the expertise of the Mayo Clinic, I went back to Puerto Rico a new person and reentered medical school. I was placed in the second semester of first year—with the class of 1970, not my original class of 1969. There was a new Chair of Physiology who eliminated all the first-year medical school laboratories, which was quite a shock to me. I had lost a year of medical school in vain—but it ended up being a blessing.

I now had a new body, a new state of mind, a new group, new friends—and they accepted me and incorporated me into their lives. This shaped my future and changed my life. God is great.

I was highly motivated and performed well. It was the best thing that could have happened to me because they never asked me what my problem was; they already knew, and I just integrated with the class like nothing had happened. In my third year of medical school, I became part of the consideration list for Alpha Omega Alpha, which is the Medical Honor Society. The first to send me a letter of congratulations was the same professor of physiology who wouldn't help me to repeat the laboratories. I didn't make Alpha Omega Alpha in medical school, but after completing my residency training, I was selected.

When I became Surgeon General, I had a reception for my medical school classes at the Puerto Rico Capitol Building. I invited members of both medical school classes I had been a part of: 1969 and 1970. The Class of 1970, though, is the class for which I feel affinity. Normalcy. To this day, I see members of both classes quite frequently.

I had a first date in medical school who took me to listen to violin concertos at the university theater. Ruggiero Ricci was playing twenty-four Paganini violin concertos. Poop ruined the date—but this time, not my poop! In the middle of the fourteenth concerto, I had to leave. My date crossed his legs and there was so much dog poop on the sole of his shoe that the odor overwhelmed me. He had to listen to the rest of that concert by himself. I hope he cleaned his shoes before his next date. He never asked me out again.

It seemed like no matter what we were doing in anatomy class, somehow the medical school cafeteria managed to give us something to eat that was pertinent to what we were dissecting. I remember that when we were dissecting the stomach and the gut, every single day there was something in there that none of us could eat. I have the feeling that the cook would talk to the anatomy teacher and plan the menus accordingly. If we were working on the liver, we had liver. It seemed like this happened all the time.

In Puerto Rico, bodies that were unclaimed for a certain number of months were turned over to the school of medicine for anatomy class. The four members of my team were in front of our cadaver, whose tag said Antonio. We were just about to put the first knife cut in when this woman entered the room screaming, "Antonio,

Antonio!" We all froze. He was removed, and we were given another cadaver. But it reminded us that we were cutting into a human and that the human had a name and belonged to his or her family. When the anatomy class finished with a cadaver, there was a proper burial for the remains. But it was freaky to have a mother come in to claim her son in the middle of class!

One of my colleagues in anatomy class was a girl whose parents were very famous. It was the day to do the dissection of the penis, and I looked over at her table. She had a rope around the base of the penis and the other part tied around her neck so that every time she would move, the penis would move so that she could dissect it. But most importantly, she never had to touch it. I wonder what specialty she did after she graduated.

I came home every weekend during medical school to study. Two years after Mami gave me the red sports car, she bought Tomas and me Triumph sports cars. By that time, my red convertible was quite leaky. I kept a towel on my lap so that when it rained, I could wipe my face and see to drive. Similarly, it was quite dented in the front by that time. Someone was always bumping into my car from the rear—causing my microscope to fly. Three times that microscope broke the windshield. Mami knew the routine and got tired of fixing the car.

Tomas got a TF 4, the "real" sports car, and I got a smaller, less sporty blue Triumph. He crashed his car one month to the day that we had been given our automotive gifts. So whose car do you think he would use Friday, Saturday, and Sunday night when he was dating? Mami would say, "He's your brother. Loan him your car." Grudgingly, I would give him the keys and my friends supplied the transportation that I needed.

This continued until one night, a policeman came to the house. Mami was very important in the lives of the local police. She praised and recognized them for their good work with many dinners and plaques. On this night, the policeman said, "Mrs. Flores, I have to tell you that we do not think it is a good idea for your daughter to be down at the beach at two or three o'clock in the morning with her legs sticking out of her car." Well, everyone in our very small town knew the blue Triumph was my car.

What? My mother went crazy—looking at me—until she realized that I didn't have a car on Friday, Saturday, and Sunday nights, and the only one who was driving my blue Triumph those nights was my brother.

Needless to say, I never had to lend him my car again, and this time Mami pushed no more. Can you imagine the gossip from people in a little town like mine? Everyone knows everybody else's business. It would have completely ruined my reputation. My stepfather ended up buying Tomas a used car (a Mustang).

CHAPTER 3

Destiny and Marriage

Roosevelt Roads was the naval station that was in Ceiba, the next town over from my hometown. During the 1960s and 1970s, many American GIs who served in Vietnam were housed there. The base commander's wife, Mrs. Moore, became my mother's friend. At the end of my second year of medical school, Mrs. Moore asked my mother if I could attend the receptions on Friday nights at the Officers Club, and my mother said yes. Mrs. Moore would get a pass for me and a friend, and we would go over to the club and have dinner and talk with some of the GIs. Mrs. Moore wanted some nice Puerto Rican girls socializing with the GIs rather than women who could be found outside the gates of the naval base.

In June of 1968, Mrs. Moore and my mother felt that I needed to meet this new doctor at the hospital at Roosevelt Roads who had just arrived from Pensacola, Florida. He had joined the Navy during the Vietnam War and been sent to Pensacola to be trained as a Navy Flight Surgeon. In his class, there was one person of Italian heritage and one person who was Latino. The Navy sent the Latino to Rome and sent Joe Novello (the Italian) to Puerto Rico! He oversaw a squadron, and he was supposed to be my blind date.

I told them, "Mami, I don't want a blind date. Your taste and Mrs. Moore's taste are not mine." I had not even decided that I wanted to have a husband. Mami said, "Well, that's your problem. But at this stage of the game, he's going to call, and he's going to try to come here and pick you up."

I was not happy. A blind date? My eye! According to Mrs. Moore, he was twenty-seven years old, single, handsome, a doctor, from Ohio, and he had just finished a full year of surgical training at Case Western Reserve. He had also graduated from the University of Michigan—and he needed to have some new friends. Truly, I thought the package was problematic: an American male, single, and a great catch at twenty-seven. I thought he could be gay. So I didn't want to meet him. To make matters worse, he called me at home and wanted to pick me up for the reception where we were supposed to meet. His voice was so deep and low. I said, "Oh my God, he's not only gay, but he sounds like a frog. I do not want to meet this man." So I said, "Don't come pick me up, I will meet you at nine o'clock." And I didn't want my neighbors (gossipy as they were) to meet this man and laugh at me behind my back.

The party started at nine p.m., and I didn't show up until midnight. It so happened that the night of the blind date was also the same night as the patron saint fiestas held at the plaza. The girls go one way, and the boys go the other. It was a good way to mingle and make new friends, keeping an eye on any new boys. The plaza was about two blocks away from the dance that Mrs. Moore and Mami had planned for that evening.

I was having fun in the plaza with my friends that evening, considerably after nine p.m. I had bought a new dress and had my hair done at the beauty shop. It was midnight when my brother, Tomas, came into the plaza. He declared that if I did not show up at the party two blocks away where this man has been waiting since nine o'clock that our mother would come to the plaza and play with my face in public. You have to know my mother to realize that she would do it.

I went to the party very grudgingly and angry beyond belief. My mother was standing at the entrance, and she alerted me that we would discuss this when we got home. I told her, "Mami, this blind date is your idea and Mrs. Moore's—not mine. Let's get this done, and point me to the monster." As I went to the ladies' room to arrange myself, Mami said, "Monster? Take a look at that table—and the man whose back is toward you surrounded by all those women—and tell me if that fits the definition of a monster."

I proceeded to fix my hair, my lipstick, and so forth and went to where this man was. I tapped him on the shoulder—an arrogant second-year medical student who did not want to be there—and proceeded to introduce myself. To my surprise, when he looked at me, my brain said, "My God, I have wasted almost three hours of time that could have been spent enjoying this blind date!" Joe wasn't what you would call super handsome, but he was very, very elegant, chic, and had a beautiful demeanor. He was in a wonderful suit; clean-cut Navy. I had never gone out with an officer before.

The liking was mutual and instantaneous. He asked me to dance. During the second dance, I thought his hand had gone too far down my back. I proceeded to remove his hand, stopped dancing, and reminded him that he was a doctor—and so was I—and that I had to be respected.

That must have been the turning point. He always said that was the thing that made him think I was different. We dated for two years, and I decided that he was the man I was going to marry. I thought since we were both going to be doctors that we would have many things in common to talk about. I felt secure around him. I thought we could get married while I was in medical school, but Joe said, "No, absolutely, no." He said he had just finished a surgical internship, and he didn't want to have that kind of life during our first year of marriage.

I wanted to be a surgeon, but Joe had other ideas. He said, "Do you want to be a married pediatrician or a single surgeon?" Joe was the oldest male in an Italian family. His father was a doctor. His mother was a nurse. His uncle was a surgeon. His aunts were nurses. His cousins were doctors. I think he didn't want to be outdone. He would be marrying a doctor, not a nurse—the first one in his family. So it made sense for him to ask me not to be a woman surgeon.

And so, of course, I became a pediatrician. And then God made me Surgeon General of the United States. Something I made sure he never forgot. So many times, we do what we need to as a couple and what is expected for the marriage to work, and we put our career on a second tier. Someday, women and men will be equals.

Joe and I knew we would be going together to the States and needed to look for residencies where we could be together. Early in our relationship, Joe wanted to be an ophthalmologist and had been accepted at Duke University. I was excited that he wanted to be an ophthalmologist. But as he tended to the GIs returning from Vietnam, he changed his mind. Why concentrate on the eyes when the body and soul were so broken? Thus, he decided he wanted to be a psychiatrist. I could not imagine such a thing because of my unfortunate experience with the Chief of Psychiatry during my medical school years. This man would put two pencils in his nose when he was giving lectures. In the back of my mind, I had always thought that psychiatrists were not well. Regardless, Joe gave up on ophthalmology and went to look for a residency in psychiatry.

We visited Cornell. We visited Case Western Reserve. And we visited the University of Michigan, where Joe had studied to be a doctor; Michigan was, at the time, probably the number one place in the US to study psychiatry. When I went for my interview there, I did not even know what football was and even less how great the university was—and I certainly had no idea what the Michigan colors were. It was summer, and I had a navy blue suit with a yellow blouse, never knowing that those were the colors of Michigan. I guess the panel was impressed. I liked the people immediately. The interviewer told me, "Well, we have already chosen the incoming intern group. At this stage, if we choose you, you will have to go to Wayne County [the city hospital] for one year, and then we will transfer you here at the beginning of your residency." I remember saying, "No, I'm either good enough to start or no good at all." Then the fax came, it said I had gotten into the University of Michigan. It is at times like this that I truly believe God had—and has—a plan for me.

* * *

I finished medical school and graduated May 29, 1970. I certainly don't remember much of my Hippocratic Oath as I was thinking of my upcoming wedding—the dress, the food, the guests, and so forth—so I just mouthed the words. The church wedding was the next day, May 30, 1970.

My little black bag of medicine said "Antonia C. Novello," when my classmates thought it should have said "Antonia Coello Flores." But I was going to marry an American, and the tradition was to take his last name. In addition, since the Navy was going to move us out of Puerto Rico, we actually got married twice. We had to get married "civilian" so that the Navy could start the proceedings with the movers. And then, of course, I am a Puerto Rican Catholic girl, so I had to get married through the church.

I think the civilian marriage was on May 13, 1970, before graduation. That same day, we attended a dinner at the Officers Club on base. We were very secretive and didn't say anything because we thought some people would talk, implying that I could be pregnant if we were getting married in a civil ceremony two weeks before the church ceremony. Then, as we are getting in the car to go to Luquillo for the civilian ceremony, we heard on the loudspeaker, "And now Dr. Novello and his bride are leaving to get married civilian." So now everyone knew. There went the privacy.

We got married civilian in the town of Luquillo with the Justice of the Peace; I don't remember much about that wedding. The judge had a dog, and that dog was huge—he was going in and out of Joe's and my legs constantly. I know it was a wedding ceremony, but I was so focused on that dog. I know I got married and that it happened because the papers exist, and that when we got to my mother's house, I told my mother that I wanted to be with Joe. She immediately said, "No, absolutely not. You already ordered the dress; you are not going to ruin everything by going with your husband today because you are not going to be the wife until the thirtieth of May!" And so, she just locked the door in his face, even though we were married. Fortunately, Joe was by that time familiar with our customs, and he went back to the base without me.

I had started taking birth control pills a month before the marriage as Joe and I had decided that we weren't going to have children while I was an intern. I knew that one side effect of birth control pills was acne and some brown stains, so I would look in the mirror every morning to see if any acne was appearing. If it had, then the whole neighborhood would think that I was having sex and I would be totally shunned. That was one thing that worried me.

Another thing that worried me was a tradition in my hometown that said if your wedding veil fell or got stuck on the tree at the entrance of the church, that meant you were not a virgin. The chapel where we would have gotten married had trees that lined the steps of the church and formed an arch overhead. I had seen many women almost bleeding through their forehead from pinning that veil to their head to make sure that it stayed on. Some must have had a hundred pins!

I had wanted to get married in Fajardo like every other nice little Puerto Rican girl of the town, but the priest had decided that May 30 was going to be his only day off. So we got married in the Chapel in the Hill at Roosevelt Roads on May 30, 1970, instead. In some ways, that was more intimate and quaint. Of course, there were a few mishaps along the way. The wife of the man who was driving me to the church was trying to apply false eyelashes and they just wouldn't go on, so we were a little late. And to make matters worse, it started raining, but for me, rain meant good luck so that was a positive sign as far as I was concerned.

It was a very pretty wedding, and everybody from the naval station was invited, including all of Joe's staff and friends. To enter the naval station, everybody had to have ID. But I was the bride, and I was not going to bring identification with me for my wedding. So the gate sentry asked me for my ID, and I said, "I don't have it with me, I am the bride." He just looked at me. And I said, "Do you think I dressed this way to get around the requirement for an ID?" He wouldn't give up. Well, Mami's housemaid was in the car behind us. She had to give me her invitation so that I could come onto the base for my own wedding.

After the wedding and during the reception, my stepfather had his hands behind his back the whole time. Everyone else greeted guests with a handshake, but he greeted like he was somebody from Japan—you know, with the bow. When the receiving line was finished, I asked him why he was not shaking hands with the guests, He said, "Because on my way here I got a flat tire." He showed me his hands and they were black, truly black.

I didn't even know if Mom and Dad Novello were coming to our wedding until the last minute when they finally arrived the day before the wedding. They weren't very happy that Joe was marrying a Puerto Rican girl; they had already broken up his previous relationship with a German girl while he had been at the University of Michigan medical school. At that time, in Lorain, Ohio, where Joe was from, the Puerto Ricans were the blue-collar people working in the steel mill who weren't middle class on the island like I was. Joe's parents wrote him a letter trying to dissuade him from marrying me. He showed me the letter; it hurt. But he tore it into many pieces and decided to go ahead with the wedding. I had asked his sister to be my maid of honor, but she declined. I have the feeling that Mom and Dad Novello wouldn't let her participate. To this day she says she feels terrible that she said no. And when she saw the bridal party—twelve bridesmaids and twelve groomsmen—coming down the church aisle with all the men in tails and the women in long dresses, I'm sure she regretted her decision.

The groomsmen were Joe's military friends, and his brother was the best man. The twelve bridesmaids included the two secretaries of the Chairman of Medicine at the medical school, my Girl Scout friends, my next-door teenage friend, a teacher, a cousin, and four friends from infancy. The flower girls were the daughter and niece of my beautician. My mother and stepfather walked me down the aisle in my designer wedding dress. After the wedding, 350 people attended the reception and dined at the Conquistador Hotel. Mami paid for everything. She even bought all my outfits for the honeymoon.

Finally, Joe and I got to our room and both of us remembered that

we hadn't eaten because we had spent all our time dancing, toasting, and saying hello to everyone at every table. So we were hungry! I called my mother from the suite and her immediate reaction was, "What's the matter, is he hurting you?" And I said, "No, Mami, I'm hungry." So she sent down two club sandwiches and two sodas, and we ate.

The morning after I was, of course, married. We were going on our honeymoon and we were to have a brunch before we left for Colombia, South America. I had told Joe, "You're not going to take

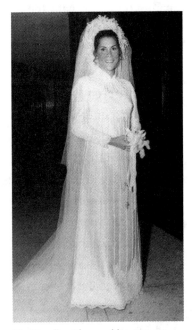

Dr. Novello at her wedding reception at the Conquistador Hotel in 1970.

me to a place that has a beach. I have lived in this all my life. I want to go somewhere else." So we went to Colombia. But the morning of the brunch, I would not lift my head. It was the embarrassment of knowing that you are married and everyone's supposition about what you have done the night before. I could not look my mother in the eye.

As luck would have it, on the first night of our honeymoon in Colombia, right outside of the hotel window there was a huge Virgin statue on the hill that I thought was looking at us. I turned beet red, closed the curtains, made the sign of the cross, and proceeded to enjoy our honeymoon. We were in Colombia for ten days and then we came back to Puerto Rico. We stayed at the Officer's Quarters until the Navy completed the move and we went to Ann Arbor, Michigan, where Joe started his residency in psychiatry, and I began my internship in pediatrics. The Navy delivered our goods late so during our first month as newlyweds we slept on air mattresses. It was not a comfortable way to start working as an intern.

Once I started earning my own salary, I was so in awe of how my mother on a $39,000 salary got a Triumph for me and my brother. How she paid for a wedding for me with 350 people and a designer gown. Paid for my medical school. She provided for me in so many ways and I honor her for that. How did she do it? I still do not know. She just did things well and never boasted.

CHAPTER 4

Off to Michigan

Joe and I lived for a while at the Bachelor's Quarters at Roosevelt Roads while our goods were arriving in Michigan. Soon thereafter, we followed, and I began my study of pediatrics as an intern.

My interns' group, maybe fourteen or fifteen of us all together, called me "Chiquita Banana" because my accent was so thick. Although I knew English, my English conversations up to that point had only been with Joe or Mrs. Moore. So, at the beginning of my internship, I was reading lips to understand what everyone was saying.

I did end up at the Wayne County hospital (the seat of Wayne County is the city of Detroit). I was supposed to be there for four months. I learned so much about pediatrics at Wayne County, for which I am quite grateful. While I was there, I used to cover the emergency room. I would tell the staff that I was going to go have dinner and then cover the ER. After dinner, I would find it full of patients, with nobody else there but me. One evening, I finally walked into a room and found all the residents playing cards and laughing about how I (the Puerto Rican intern) was taking care of the patients. I reported them. Suddenly, there was more respect. I continued to take care of all my patients and more than my share. One day the Chief of Pediatrics of Wayne County came to me and said, "It's time for you to go home." I had just admitted fourteen patients, and I protested that there were more patients to see. He said there would always be more patients and that it was time for me to go home.

Well, to my surprise, I won the Intern of the Year award. People said things like, "Although she speaks English, she always looks at your lips." "She's always available to help you." "She doesn't shy away from seeing more patients." "She's funny and at the same time helpful." At the University of Michigan, when you get the Intern of the Year award, you don't get a plaque. You get a chamber pot. A ceramic chamber pot. I was very reticent about taking this award, thinking maybe it was because I took so much crap. But then I looked at the names on the rim and I felt that they walked on water. So, I decided, "Give me the chamber pot. I don't care." I called Mami, and I said, "Mami, I am Intern of the Year of the University of Michigan Class of seventy–seventy-one." She said, "And, how is your plaque?" I said, "No, no, no. They gave me a chamber pot." She said, "What?" I said, "Yes, they gave me a chamber pot." And she said, "Those 'gringos' gave you a chamber pot when you're good? Make sure you don't call me when you're bad." I have no idea what she thought they would give me if I misbehaved. When I looked at the rim of the chamber pot I understood that this was an important award. The people whose names were on the rim—and mine is there now too—became Chief Residents, great members of the community, and great physicians. I would never have dreamed that a chamber pot award would take me so far.

When we lived in Michigan, we visited Mom and Dad Novello about once a month in Lorain, Ohio. I decided to go in their lives with a clean slate. I was not going to remind them of what they thought about me in the letter. They needed to get to know me personally. I was going to be the best daughter-in-law that I could.

At the end of Mom and Dad Novellos' lives, even though Joe and I were divorced, I was almost like the resident doctor in the house. When I lived in Albany, New York, I would fly in constantly if Mom or Dad had a problem. And I was always taking responsibility because at that point Joe had a new girlfriend who was occupying his time. At the end of Mom Novello's life, she said she wanted to make sure that she saw her family before she died, so I had a picture made—everyone in the family was there in that picture but me. When she was in hospice and the nurse told me she was dying and trying to say good-bye, I ran and got the picture and put it in front of her face so that she could see the whole family. When she died, I was the only family member in the room. My sister-in-law was outside with her car as she had been having problems with her phone battery. I will never be able to forget that moment because when my sister-in-law walked into the room, I said, "Mom just died." And she said, "Oh, come on. Mom is always dying—you know what I mean?" We had thought she was dying the month before, so the whole family was called in, but she didn't die. I said, "No, this time it is real." It broke my heart how much she cried. At Mom's funeral, I had a place of honor even though Joe was there with his girlfriend.

In the end, I was no longer the Puerto Rican, I was the one who was helpful. I had started the relationship on the right foot—I went in as a lady first. And behaved as one until the end.

While I was an intern, I became very good at physical exams and catching veins. This is because of what happened with my leukemia patients. First, I had Keith. Keith was seven years old and had rhabdomyosarcoma of the prostate. He was very skinny and very sickly, and I knew that with his tumor he was going to die. I tried to do the very best job I could for him until he was gone. Then I inherited a little girl of no more than six. I needed to administer her che-

"That was when I realized that you do not make promises you cannot keep."

motherapy, and I told her, "This is not going to hurt you, I am going to get your vein on the first try." I missed. She looked at me and she had a tear coming out of her eye, which made me more nervous as I tried once more. I missed again. She slapped me in the face.

That was when I realized that you do not make promises you cannot keep, especially for sick children. The patients need to be able to trust you. I needed more experience. I promised what I

"Underpromise and overdeliver. A lesson that I learned over and over."

could not deliver. The cockiness of being the doctor was now replaced with my feeling awful. And so I became a better doctor because I had failed that little girl who slapped me in the face.

From that moment on, I practiced, and I practiced, and I practiced. It got to the point in the internship that if there was ever a problem with catching a vein, I was called.

My fellow interns would laugh at me because I was different, but they were fond of me. Still, I learned I needed to always do better—underpromise and overdeliver. A lesson that I learned over and over.

As I said, I read lips, as that was the best way for me to learn conversational English. I learned that the best people to know immediately were the nurse in the unit and, more than anything, the secretary, because that way you got your lab tests done before anybody else. They cared for you because you cared for them. A very important lesson to have learned.

I also had a little boy named Paul. He was so sad-looking. I would sneak him out of the hospital once a week while he was hospitalized. I would make dinner for him at home. I knew that he was not going to make it. Joe and I became very fond of Paul. One day I was speaking with his nurses, and I told them that I thought it would be very good for Paul to have a puppy. They said, "Well, Dr. Novello, there are so many allergic children on the ward." But I said, "He's in a single room. Is there any way we could sneak the puppy in and hide it so that no one sees it? I think it would be wonderful for Paul as he is so depressed." So they looked the other way, and I bought him a puppy. After I paid for that puppy, my purse disappeared. And I remember that I talked to God, and I said, "God, if I did a good deed, why do I have to lose everything and start anew getting my license and all that stuff?" And you won't believe it, but the morning after the purse—with no money—was found in one of the hospital mailboxes. I was pleased that God heard me and pleased that Paul had his puppy. No more than a month later, Paul was dead. The dog died soon thereafter. I was told they were buried together.

At the Wayne County Hospital, you learn about almost every aspect of medicine because of the neighborhood and the variety of diseases encountered there. As the pediatrician, I was once called because a man had shot his wife, who was nine months pregnant, and then killed himself. The baby was born by Caesarian section and he was alive. As I was looking at the baby, I was thinking, *God, this baby has no father, this baby has no mother, what is going to happen with him?* You have to do what you have to do. That baby needed to be intubated to deliver oxygen. And, on top of everything else, the electricity went out. So, for eight hours, I delivered oxygen manually to this baby using a technique called "bagging." Using a bag, I pushed air and oxygen into his lungs. The baby was transferred to the University of Michigan but did not survive long-term, despite all our efforts. God knew best.

One day when I was on call for the ER, a woman came in who must have weighed three hundred pounds or more. She was in pain. She was so large that they had to take the X-rays in quadrants until they were able to have a complete one. To everyone's amazement, including hers, she was pregnant and in labor. Nobody had even contemplated that outcome—they thought gall bladder or appendix. I was called: "Will the pediatrician please come to the delivery room?" I went, and she had a baby. We asked her if anyone accompanied her to the ER. She said yes and gave us his name. This rather skinny, small man answered when I asked for him, and he said he did accompany the woman. He asked if everything was okay with her. I said, "Well I have good news for you. She just had a baby." And the next thing I know, this guy fainted in front of me. I had never seen a couple happier with such unexpected news.

There was a tremendous drug crisis in the 1970s. Many of the babies born in the hospital were shaky as they were in withdrawal from cocaine or whatever the mother was taking. One baby was very shaky, and before we administered medication, the resident told me I needed to go talk to the mother and ask her if she was doing drugs or had a history of drug use. This was very early in my internship, and so I did what I was told. I went and asked the mother if she had been doing drugs. The woman, probably one and a half times my size, stood up, looked at me, and said, "That is exactly what my husband asked before I killed him." I had never run so fast in my life. I am pretty sure the resident knew that was going to happen and sent me there as a joke. But I certainly got savvier after that about what and to whom I asked.

While an intern, I was invited to a pool party. Another guest and I arrived at the front door to ring the doorbell at the same time. I was wearing a bathing suit that came with a skirt to match and a matching turban that I wore on my head. I thought I looked like a movie star. The woman on my right was wearing a long formal gown, pearls, and a tiara. And I thought, *God, one of us has read the invitation incorrectly and if it is me, I am going to die.* The door opened and the host was wearing a sarong with a bathing suit and skirt. Why was the woman dressed formally for a pool party? I later learned that she was going to the opera, but she wanted to make an appearance at the pool party first. She had a drink and off she went to the opera.

Our Chief of Pediatrics, Dr. William Oliver, was from Georgia. He had a crew cut and a very strong personality. Every Friday we had grand rounds where every patient was presented to him by the intern on call. Dr. Oliver used to stand with his legs in an open stance during those grand rounds. One Friday, a little kid, maybe four years old, on a tricycle, ran right through his legs, probably hit a testicle, and the man's voice didn't even change. He never even blinked.

As luck would have it, Dr. Oliver was in Venezuela on the day of his twenty-fifth wedding anniversary, so Joe and I went to visit with his wife, Marguerite. Dr. Oliver was investigating new strands of bacteria and had named one of them for her. She said that she never thought that for her twenty-fifth anniversary, she would be spending it with Toni and Joe Novello, and that on top of that an *E. coli* bacteria was going to be named for her. What a gift!

When I became Surgeon General in 1990, Joe arranged a special dinner for those people who were most dear in our lives. Dr. Oliver and Marguerite were among them. During coffee and dessert, Joe asked if anyone wanted to stand up and say a few words. Dr. Oliver stood up and said he wanted to state publicly that when my application came to the University of Michigan for pediatrics, he was very reluctant to have me admitted to the internship group. This was because, at the time, he felt only Americans should come straight into the internships, and my being Puerto Rican wasn't the same. In addition, he didn't like the picture that my university sent— one in which I was wearing pearls and a little white rabbit stole. He now believed that it would have been a mistake for the University of Michigan not to admit me due to such prejudice. After all, I had won the Intern of the Year and was now the Surgeon General of the United States. He didn't know when Michigan would have another one like me, but he was so proud that he helped me come on board. By this time, Joe and I were sitting there with our mouths wide open. Who knew that this proud man would open up his heart so publicly in front of a group who were basically strangers to him?

* * *

I suspected that Joe had been unfaithful during our first year of marriage while I was doing my internship. This would have been with the secretary in charge of typing his first book. I was on the elevator with a psychiatrist one day, and he asked me, "When is this book going to be over? I really want my wife to be home earlier." I had not been paying attention because I was so busy doing my internship. All I wanted was time to sleep, time to cook, and then go to bed. So one day, I walked into my house, locked the door very softly, and heard Joe talking on the phone with someone while sitting on the bed with his legs crossed. He looked almost like you see teenagers talking on the phone in the movies. I thought something was happening, but I was too busy to give any time to it. I also believed that if I brought it up, he would deny it.

From the day I met Joseph, every month there would be a pink envelope that arrived at his office and another one that came to the house. Those pink envelopes were from the German girlfriend he had had when he was at the University of Michigan. Envelopes were still arriving monthly at the time of our divorce. Joe never went to Germany to visit his old girlfriend, and he did not marry the woman with whom he had had an affair for twenty years while we were married either. Joe is a good man. I believe that we got married at the right time for the right reasons. But I always wondered if he had been cheated out of marrying and being in love with the writer of those letters in the pink envelopes.

Joe and I lived in an apartment complex while I was an intern. A new intern group came after us, and one of the new interns and his wife became our next-door neighbors. I wanted to welcome them to the complex and to the university so I prepared some chicken soup for them. When the wife opened the door, she thanked me but said that they kept kosher and so they wouldn't be able to accept my soup. What does a Puerto Rican girl know about kosher? I thought it meant something about culturing the bacteria. By the time we left the complex, we had become very good friends and we could share a laugh about the incident.

* * *

Joe and I decided not to try and have children during the first year of my residency. He thought ER exposure might result in my picking up an infection, so we started trying in my second year, but I did not get pregnant.

I started doing the tests to determine fertility. The hysterosalpingogram evaluates your Fallopian tubes with X-rays and dye to determine if they are open. Three women, including me, were in the room having the test done at the same time with three different cameras showing up on three different screens. I was in the middle. I was looking at all the screens—the one on the left showed open Fallopian tubes. The one on my right showed open Fallopian tubes. My dye did not go all the way up. The doctor said he was going to put more dye in to see if there was a blockage. Still the dye did not move through my Fallopian tubes for the second time.

This was at the University of Michigan, and the doctor said he would need to request my records. Since they were in Spanish, and I was the only one who could read Spanish, I would need to read and translate the notes from my operations. The records from Teacher's Hospital arrived, and I read the operative note from the surgery in Puerto Rico when I was eighteen. The pathology report said, "presence of a cut Fallopian tube in the operative field, presence of a dermoid tumor, remnants of abscess formation in (R) inguinal area, where second Fallopian tube was found." No one ever told me of all those findings; I had to discover them by reading my own medical records in Spanish during my second year of residency.

When I had my surgery in Puerto Rico, I had just completed my sophomore year in natural sciences at the University of Puerto Rico. I was not stupid. I was just sick. And this doctor whom I had trusted with my life and future never told me the complications of my surgery— never told me he had cut one of my Fallopian tubes. Never told me a word—even though he saw me for almost nine months during my rectal dilatation visits! Was this medicine as people feel it should be?

Joe and I cried. We were devastated. A cardiac surgeon should not be doing intestinal surgery. Joe really wanted to sue, but ten years had passed, and we felt that the statute of limitations had expired.

"I was going to be empathetic with my patients."

This discovery when I was twenty-eight years old hardened my resolve. I would absolutely be better than those who could have ruined my life and future. I would absolutely be the opposite of those who kept me in the dark. I would never be like *him*:

- I was going to be a better doctor.
- I was never going to keep my patients in the dark.
- I was going to be a great communicator.
- I was going to be empathetic with my patients.
- I would not drop anyone for lack of payments or for personal reasons.

I only saw the cardiac doctor one more time in my life. In 1990, I won the Pediatrician of the Year Award from the Ronald McDonald Foundation. The prize included $100,000 that was to be donated to a not-for-profit organization. I chose to donate it to the Teacher's Hospital of Puerto Rico. They created an area for mammograms that was named for my mother, and they wanted me to come and inaugurate it. Unfortunately, I did not know that that cardiac doctor's family member was the doctor in charge of the mammogram facility. And more unfortunately, he was invited. He went to the podium and said, "Everything she is she owes it to me." I was furious and I left the podium.

How dare he say that all I am I owe to him? But yes, in a way, it is true. I became a better doctor than him because I had to grow up fast, because of his mistakes and lack of truth and transparency. I still don't know if I can ever forgive him.

My mother was there with me, and she was going crazy. "What kind of behavior is this? How dare you move out of there when they are introducing you!" I said, "Mami, if I stayed there, I would have slapped him, so please don't let me be in his presence." I had never shared with Mami all the complications and other issues from my surgery. This was the first time that she understood. I could not face him as an adult—and now he is dead, and I don't have to face him at all, ever again. I certainly learned, though, the importance of a second opinion, which I never had. A human being taking care of human beings needs more transparency.

Once we learned that I couldn't have children, Joe and I decided to pursue adoption. We put ourselves into Catholic Charities with one requirement—we wanted a child that had either some Latin blood or some Italian blood. We waited close to five years and the child we were looking for was never found. Would it be half Hispanic or half Italian? We were contacted about adopting disabled children but were not interested in pursuing that option. Joe had decided that when the baby came, one way or the other, I would have to stop my practice. I was agreeable; I had no problems with that. We even looked at adoption possibilities in Europe, in Latin America, and in Canada. But a child never came.

* * *

I had decided at the time of Mami Loli's death during my medical school years that no one would suffer from kidney disease if I could help it. Thus, I decided to take a fellowship in kidney disease after I had completed my residency. I was sent to do work in the dialysis unit. All the other University of Michigan fellows had been sent to Vietnam because they were part of the Berry Plan. So there I was in the pediatric nephrology unit working with the adult nephrology team. As it happened, I was also needed in the adult nephrology branch, so I ended up getting double training in pediatric and adult nephrology.

Then, ironically, I got acute pyelonephritis, which is a huge inflammation of the kidneys, during my fellowship. I was hospitalized and quite sick. It gave me tremendous insight into how my nephrology patients felt and thus how I needed to treat them. I read my chart after I was discharged and saw that I had been "unable to eat." How could I? At that time, IV fluids were administered while your hand was extended with tape on a flat board. I am right-handed and it was my right hand.

There were three fellows in adult nephrology and one in pediatric nephrology—four of us all together. And I was always called Toni Novello. When graduation day came for my fellowship, I decided to wear a pink suit. I think that was the first time that the wives of the other three realized that I was a woman, that "Toni Novello" wasn't a man. All those times, we four fellows spent twenty-four hours on call. I think the wives were in shock. But Toni was dressed in pink—and was an elegant woman. Surprise! Thank God I was married.

I really believe that being at the University of Michigan was for me the right university at the right time. It opened my eyes and opened my future. In 1991, when the School of Public Health at the University of Michigan celebrated its fiftieth anniversary, Sanjay Gupta, a neurosurgeon and chief medical correspondent for CNN, and I were some of the alums asked to celebrate through words our life at Michigan. The university never forgot the little girl from Puerto Rico, and the little girl from Puerto Rico never forgot the University of Michigan. Truth be known, my heart will always belong to the University of Michigan.

CHAPTER 5

Washington, D.C., Beckons

In 1972, when research money dried up under President Richard Nixon, Joe and I decided to leave Michigan. Joe was hired at what was then called the Psychiatry Institute of Washington, D.C., as a partner. I went to Georgetown University as a second-year fellow in pediatric nephrology.

Georgetown was very interested in doing organ transplants for children. While I was there, we did the first transplantations of kidneys in adolescents. We did many transplants, and I finished my fellowship working every other night, every other weekend on call. While I was at Georgetown, some of my patients' parents became lifetime friends.

At one point, my favorite patient went into cardiac arrest at age twelve and died. He had the disease cystinosis, and transplants were not yet readily available. I remember that I worked on him for a long time until his mother came and told me, "You can let him go. I understand what you're doing, but you can let him go." To this day, she is one of my very best friends. When her second son developed the same renal disease—which was congenital and genetic—like his brother, I told her, "We can either be friends or I can be your doctor, but I cannot be both." I cannot go through this again. We became friends. The second son had a transplant using his mother's kidney, became a doctor, and lived to be in his forties. This was despite doctors who told him he wasn't going to make it. He used to tell me, "I have to make it. I have to show that even those of us with disabilities can conquer them and be somebody." Like me, he wanted to overcome the challenges, the dismissive people, to prove people wrong. He was not a tall man and he had difficulty speaking because of his disease. But he became a very good primary care doctor. When he graduated from medical school in upstate New York, I was the commencement speaker. When he died, I spoke at his funeral. Never underestimate those who want to be somebody in spite of tremendous odds.

During the time I was at Georgetown, one of the Saudi Arabian princesses came to do her internship at the university. I was quite fond of her, both because she came from a different country and because she had Potts disease—she must have had tuberculosis when she was a child—which caused a hunchback and deformed bones. At one point in her internship, she decided to bring her mother and her sister to go with her on a trip to Disney World. The Chief of Pediatrics decided that I would accompany the family on the trip. I learned a lot about different values and cultural differences on this trip.

I took the princess, her mother, and her sister to Disney World and then to Miami Beach. They wanted to stay at Disney World from the moment it opened until the moment it closed. We used every single opportunity to enjoy the rides and ourselves. We closed Disney every night. Since they had paid for the privilege of attending, they wanted to enjoy every penny spent.

> "Never underestimate those who want to be somebody in spite of tremendous odds."

We then went to Miami Beach and stayed in the Fontainebleau hotel—our rooms were connected by a door. I believe the hotel staff played a little joke on the Arab princess and her family when they called on the phone and requested that a movie be played in their room. I heard what I think was a porno movie (*Deep Throat*) in their room. I went in, and the three of them were there in the room, glued to the television. The mother said something along the lines of "Just look and see, watch him, now he will steal her purse." I accompanied no one on trips after that unless I knew them well.

When the princess got her internship diploma, we had to redo it and issue her a new one. This is because the standard diploma says Dr. So-and-So has served her internship at Georgetown University. She said that she couldn't take that diploma back to Saudi Arabia, however, because no Saudi serves anyone. So we fixed it and on she went.

After being on call every other night and every other week-end for two years, I thought I needed six months in which I didn't see human beings. I just wanted to do what I wanted. But within a month, I was so bored I wanted to die. So on Fridays, I went to work with a pediatric doctor in his private practice. He would give me his most difficult patients of the week to see on Friday afternoons. One patient had come the day before to see the doctor and then came again to see me on Friday afternoon. I asked the mother if her son's condition had changed since the day before. She said, "No I just brought him because I thought you probably can give me a different opinion." Well, I did a complete medical school examination. To my amazement, I realized that his liver was on top of his pelvis. I immediately got him transferred to the ER because I knew that something was very wrong with this child. He was diagnosed with acute leukemia. The doctor with whom I was working and who had missed the diagnosis went to see the child that night, charging $200 for a special visit. I, however, was getting $11 for everything that I did for a patient. That day, I quit the practice. I could not work for someone who had no shame and still charged for his mistakes.

When it was time to take my boards in pediatrics, I said to my husband, "Joseph, should I kill myself studying for these boards when I am going to be always working in government jobs and they are not necessary for employment?" Joe said, "Go ahead and take your boards because one day somebody will use the absence of them as an excuse to not give you the job you deserve." I took them, and I passed.

I became a pediatrician and worked in the Chief of Pediatric's practice at Fairfax Hospital (today it is Inova), an important hospital in northern Virginia. He would pay me 35 percent of my consultations and would not let me participate in a percentage of the laboratory tests, although I ordered most of them and the lab belonged to him. He would also not let me go and see patients at night. I thought it was very gentlemanly of him until I realized the amount of money he was making from those visits—none of which was shared with me. My fee for a consult ranged from $10 to $15. His fee for the after-hours visits was $200. Eventually, he asked me to buy his practice—eighteen beds, three nurses, five rooms, and a huge mortgage. This was during the time that I had a legal separation from Joe, and I did not want to incur any major debt. At about the same time, a woman came in with a newborn and after a complete examination, I realized that the baby was born totally blind. I was frustrated, sad, and devastated because the baby had been seen in the practice before and had not been diagnosed as blind. I decided to leave that practice as well and not buy it. When the pediatrician cries more than the parents, it's time to go.

* * *

In 1977, after seven years of marriage, Joe and I were legally separated for a year. I had noticed that Joe was becoming colder and colder—and more distant. One night I made dinner as usual, but when he arrived home Joe said he had already eaten. On a whim, I asked him who he had eaten with, and he mentioned the name of a friend. I said, "That's odd. That friend just called you to see where you were." Then Joe became very nervous, and that is when I thought something untoward was happening. I believed that he was seeing other women. I just could not prove it. But I did remember many phone calls and many hang ups when I answered. Being caught, with my trust shattered, we opted for a legal separation.

He stayed at our house, while I moved into an apartment. He provided me with $350 per month, and I was able to get my mail at our home every Sunday as provided for by the separation agreement. One Sunday, I put my house key in the lock and opened the door to go get my mail. I saw a shadow in front of my eyes. Every woman in the world thinks about what she would do if she found her husband cheating on her. Well, the moment arrived and I did not grab the other woman by the hair and strangle her on the spot, though God knows I thought about it. Instead, I decided to take the high road. I was still the wife and considered myself the lady of that house, so I turned around, closed the door, and left. I could hear Joe coming down the steps from the second floor saying, "Toni, no, Toni, no." But I did see a woman in a long gown going to the lower part of the house. Devastated, I went back to my apartment, lay down on the sofa, and stared at the ceiling for a long time. Hours later, there was a note from Joe under the door of my apartment saying, "Please remember, you are the only one I love." I cannot understand men, and worse, Joe in particular.

The very first time that I had my own credit card was when we were legally separated. All my checks had previously gone to Joe. I was a doctor, but I was not an independent woman. So I was petrified at the thought of moving in the world on my own when I moved into that apartment for a year. I was a protected child from Puerto Rico. Unknowingly, in his own way, Joe always pushed me to be better but never to be equal.

I felt very tired during the separation, but I still worked at the clinic every day. I had a hemoglobin of five and my belly was getting big. I had a D&C at Georgetown University and a fibroma, around two to three pounds, was diagnosed. Joe and I decided to go to the Mayo Clinic. When I went to the Mayo Clinic it was my hope that when they opened me up to take out the fibroma that something could be done to "fix me up"—anything to make me whole again so that I could get pregnant. They told me they would do everything possible. But when I woke up from the anesthesia, I learned that they had not been able to fix anything—and instead I came out with a complete hysterectomy. They left me with my ovaries because I was so young. Joe left the day after the surgery and I was left alone to dwell with my emptiness. So much for having a psychiatrist for a husband. One week after the surgery he returned and picked me up.

I have always contrasted Joe's behavior toward me and my fibroma surgery with his behavior when our cat, Niki, had her hysterectomy. Joe took one whole day to investigate the CV of the veterinarian who was doing Niki's surgery. Then he proceeded to take a full day off from his practice to tend to her while she was recovering. *Wow!* It is at times like that that I wish I had been Niki.

While we were legally separated and living apart, we finally had the long-awaited call from the Catholic Charities adoption agency—Joe was ecstatic. I was not. I refused the baby that was offered after five years of waiting for the miracle. Something in my heart made me say no—and God knows I wanted to say yes. But I knew that babies are not bandages for bad marriages or relationships. I knew that if I had accepted the baby, the economic maintenance would have been Joe's, but the true responsibility would have been all mine. As it was, Joe had decided that it would be my career that would have to change to accommodate a baby: half-time, three days a week—the rest was baby time. The timing was wrong, and the decision was right. The marriage needed fixing, but this baby was not to be used for fixing it. So by saying no, I became the mother of none—but the pediatrician of many. A day does not go by that I wish I could know what happened to that baby girl.

During the entire separation, Joe continued to date, although he was always in his own way watching over me. I went back with him after the separation year because I didn't know where else to go. I had no uterus, no hope of being a mother, no desire to go through the adoption process again. I had no real marriage. I was desolate, lonely, depressed. I came back also because I hoped he had learned his lesson regarding infidelity and getting caught. When I walked into our bedroom, all I could think was, *How many women have enjoyed the privacy of my bed?* All those questions and memories were not helpful to my recovery—of finding my "center."

As I looked around, I saw that the bedroom was different from the one I had left. It now had large blue furniture—extremely masculine—with very deep blue curtains as well. I thought it was probably the taste of the decorator he had hired before I left. My feelings were many. My depression hidden. But I thought, *This is not my house—but there is no other place I can go.* The contract for my rental was over, so I did what survival is all about. I became submissive with my demeanor and body language—I was almost thanking Joe for taking me back—silently believing that I had been the one who failed.

It was an awful time in my life. I started integrating slowly. I took half of the closet that used to be mine, and I begged in a subtle way for acceptance. Mind you, I wanted this marriage to work. But God—it seemed it depended mostly on me. I still wonder if Joe realized the sacrifices I made to be able to forget the rejections, the lack of empathy regarding adoption—all the offenses—and just work on being accepted back—as if all the bad things that happened in our marriage were only my fault.

* * *

During the time I was at the pediatrics practice at Fairfax Hospital, every Wednesday afternoon I noticed a man who came in dressed in a white uniform. I asked him about the uniform and what he was doing in the practice. He said he was a doctor, a member of the Public Health Service (PHS) and that as part of the PHS you have twenty hours a month to do whatever practice you were trained in. That was when I decided that I wanted to be part of the Public Health Service:

medicine and uniform—that was for me. I had always dreamed of myself as a graduate of one of the military schools. In the absence of that, the PHS was the next best choice for me.

Before joining the PHS, however, I tried to work as a pediatric nephrologist at Bethesda Naval Hospital since I was now fully certified, had married a naval officer, and the job was being advertised. I applied for the job and went in for my interview. To my amazement, when I arrived, the Captain with whom I was interviewing put his feet up on his desk, took out a copy of the *Washington Post*, and proceeded to read it. Somehow, he must have remembered that I was there waiting for some sort of communication regarding the job. At that time, he moved the paper away from his face, looked at me, and said, "Didn't you hear? We are looking for a few good men."

I went blank. This was the first time in my life that I had been treated with such disrespect. When I was about to let him have a piece of my mind, his secretary walked into the room and told me, "Honey, if you really want to join the Navy and get this job, don't listen to jerks like this—go to the Navy Bureau and apply."

I left in a daze—frustrated, angry, and in disbelief. Why had I let this obvious jerk treat me this way? I crossed Wisconsin Avenue, and there was the National Institutes of Health. I applied to join the Public Health Service that day to become a US Public Health Service Lieutenant officer, not a Naval officer.

I was one of three doctors who applied to join the Public Health Service that day—and the only one who told the truth on the application. Joe and I had been seeing a counselor for marital issues. One of the questions on the application asked if there had been any psychological visits or problems in the recent past. I assumed marital counseling fit into that category, and so I answered yes.

The woman doctor representing the Public Health Service then told me that I could not join because I had seen a psychologist. Even worse, she next told me that if the psychological visit didn't keep me out of the PHS, my congenital megacolon and its complications would. I went ballistic. I told her that I had overcome the congenital megacolon and all its complications, and she was not going to deny me this opportunity and set me back in time—especially since all those years of pain and other issues were behind me and were under control. I sent a formal letter of complaint and followed it up with a letter from the President of the American Psychiatric Association who had helped Joe and me when we needed counseling. The response to my complaint was fast and swift. I was then allowed to join the PHS as I had wanted. I was assigned to the NIH.

As for the other two doctors who applied that same day? Both were hired. One had ulcerative colitis and the other had problems with his liver, but neither disclosed their issue on their application so they didn't have to fight for the job like I did. I still believe I did the right thing. Then—and even now—it seems that psychological or mental issues and their aftermath are perceived to be worse problems than physical ones. The tolerance is minimal for the former and blind for the latter. It seems that in medicine our vulnerabilities are perceived as liabilities.

Once I had a job at the NIH, my mental state improved. I had a job that used my medical skills and my knowledge of nephrology. I resolved that I would participate more in making my marriage work, and I was ready for a new chapter in my life.

During my first years at the NIH, I worked as a contracting officer, a stint that was followed by time as a grants management officer. I then became Executive Secretary reviewing all the grants related to kidneys and bones in the US. Later, I became Deputy Director of the National Institute for Child Health and Human Development.

In those early years at the NIH, I did not regularly wear my uniform. This was because the Director of the NIH was not enamored with the Public Health Service. In fact, the first time I wore my uniform when I went to see Dr. C. Everett Koop, his assistant told me that

I smelled like mothballs. I had meetings with the NIH director every Wednesday, and I kept a black jacket in my office that I would wear instead of the black jacket of my uniform to attend those meetings. Later, Dr. Koop, the Surgeon General at the time, recommended me to chair the Revitalization Task Force to reevaluate ranks and salaries of PHS officers. After the Task Force results were published, I was able to recognize the officers of the Public Health Service serving at NIH—particularly the ones in the hospital and research system—with the ranks and salaries they truly merited. This allowed these officers to be acknowledged as the excellent researchers they were at the prestigious NIH.

The relationship between NIH and the Public Health Service had not been good in a while. When that Director had taken office, one of the first things he did was remove the Public Health anchor at the entrance of the NIH. During the Vietnam War, the PHS was one of the agencies that people joined to avoid military service. This led to the PHS officers being called the "yellow jackets" instead of getting the respect they deserved. But the Public Health Service worked to get that respect back—both with research and through the lives saved at the hospitals they staffed, including Walter Reed.

When I was Executive Secretary at the Division of Grants Review, all the other reviewers that I worked with had PhDs; I was the only MD. I didn't tell anyone because my previous boss told me that all I had to know to be qualified for the job was how to write. But eventually, people discovered that I was an MD, and those who were sick would come to me with sore throats and all other kinds of ailments.

The process for reviewing grants involved three-day meetings every three months with the top doctors in the country who had been selected to be grant reviewers. Just being in their presence was very engaging. I made sure I chose the best reviewers for my bone and kidney subdivision, and that helped quite a bit. When my group declared that a grant would be paid, the recipients knew that it had been reviewed by the best in their scientific field. That also worked well for me because when it came time for me to have letters of recommendation, the reviewers in the group were the ones who wrote them. When you are in the right place at the right time with the right preparation, nothing can stop you.

Then I would compile what happened at the meeting so that doctors at the universities who had submitted the grants could start doing the approved work. This required writing what was called the "pink slip." These pink slips had to be in the hands of universities and the principal investigator within thirty working days. Many of my colleagues would take most of those thirty days to write their reports. But I used to do them all over one weekend so I could study for my master's degree classes at Johns Hopkins. One of my colleagues came to me and said that I was putting them all to shame because I was writing my reports too quickly.

We used to have at least one hundred proposals to review, so I not only had to send them to the regular members of the review team—sometimes I would also have to look to consultants for assistance when the proposal was outside the realm of my team's expertise. Occasionally, one of the things that happened during the process was the need to stop the review. If there was ever a hint that a grant proposal was going to be disapproved or given a bad score—because it was competing for the same research dollars as was one of the reviewers—I would stop the review and call for a site visit. This was a maneuver totally under my control, and it meant that the grant in question had a chance of surviving because I would oversee choosing the new reviewers. I only had to employ this tactic about three times until the group realized that a bad review due to competitive research was not allowed in my section. Also, at

> **"When you are in the right place at the right time with the right preparation, nothing can stop you."**

the end of the review cycle, I let the Chairman know how many of the total one hundred were approved and how many were not.

With time, I thought I was going to be selected as Director of a subsection of review, but one of the older members of the executive secretariat who was about a year away from retirement was selected instead as it was exactly what he wanted before he retired. It was devastating for me not to be selected to be the subsection chief, but it taught me patience. It was not that I was not able to do the job. I learned that sometimes loyalty to your peer's service becomes paramount.

During my tenure as Executive Secretary of grants review, I earned my master's degree in public health from Johns Hopkins. The NIH management said that as long as I paid for it, I could do it, so I did. Most people taking a master's degree in public health choose to emphasize either biostatistics or epidemiology. But I got interested in government and health administration and ended up taking my master's in health services administration. A class in health and government during my master's course truly changed my life and was the reason I decided I wanted to do a Congressional Fellowship.

* * *

I quickly realized that even if government was my world, I still knew very little about it. I decided that being assigned to Congress could help me gain additional experience and knowledge. In addition, I wanted only to work with a committee responsible for matters of health. So the choice would have been to work with either Senator Ted Kennedy (D-MA) or Senator Orrin Hatch (R-UT), depending on which party was in control at the time. The committee was the US Senate Committee on Health, and Senator Hatch had become the chair of that committee during my stint.

Luckily, my neighbors happened to be Mormons who were very active in the church, and they knew Senator Hatch by first name.

They recommended me, and he took me on for six months. After that time, I continued to work for the Senator even though I had forgotten to ask permission from the PHS. As it happened, in one of the hearings, members of the Public Health Service saw me sitting behind the Senator and told me that it was time for me to come back to the NIH. I was quite embarrassed for having committed such a political faux pas. Needless to say, I asked the PHS for permission to extend my six-month fellowship, and it was granted. The Senator kept me for eighteen months rather than six after that.

One of the biggest projects that we worked on was cigarette labels (the ones saying that smoking is dangerous to your health). The cigarette labeling was very hard fought; the people from the cigarette industry thought the idea of labeling cigarettes was useless. The industry was ignoring smoking among children and pregnant women as well. No one was really paying attention to the fact that the labels should be targeted to include women and children, so I fought very hard for that one.

Another significant effort was the 1984 National Organ Transplant Act. This act established a framework for how organ transplants were to be utilized and set up a nationwide matching system. It also outlawed private payments for organs to be used in transplants outside of the transplant list.

Through both of these efforts and others during my time with Senator Hatch, I learned to be a team player and to leave my ego at the door. The Senator gets the accolades, but we the team got to see the work accomplished.

During those eighteen months, Senator Hatch tore his Achilles tendon, and during his recovery, he needed support hose. I was asked to procure them for him, and somehow, twice, I came back with the wrong size—the Senator put them on and both times they fell down. It looked for a time that the reason he was going to remember me was because of my failure to get the right size support hose!

Finally, as he was putting on the support hose, I looked at his legs—they were tall and lanky and skinny. So the third time I was sent out, I went to the hospital section where they sell the hose. I looked at one of the orderlies and I said, "Can I look at your legs please?" He pulled up his pants so I could see his legs, and I saw that they were the same size as Senator Hatch's. I asked him what size socks he wore, bought that size, and when I gave them to Senator Hatch, this time, they stuck and didn't fall down. I said, "Thank you, God, for orderlies with skinny legs."

During my time with the Senator, I learned that he really liked short memos that included everything he needed in half a page: What's the purpose? How many people will be saved or damaged because of the action you want to do? What is the prospective cost to the budget? How many people will be able to take advantage of this? And what kind of press will be covering this? If you went longer than half a page, there was no reason to bother writing it because neither the Chief of Staff nor the Senator would read it—he had so many things competing for his attention. I learned so much about formatting and writing during those eighteen months.

I believe that this eighteen-month fellowship was key to my career advancement. There were four fellows serving on the Health Committee under Senator Hatch. One became the Assistant Secretary for Legislation at the Department of Health and Human Services (HHS). David Sundwall became the administrator of the Health Resources and Services Administration (HRSA). David Kessler became the Commissioner of the Food and Drug Administration. And I became the United States Surgeon General. Quite a class of fellows it was. All I learned was not in kindergarten. Instead, I learned so much during the eighteen months of my fellowship and I have used it all throughout my career.

* * *

When I served as Executive Secretary reviewing all the grants for kidney and bone diseases at the NIH, my boss was looking for a job change and gave me his résumé. He was planning to speak about how to write a grant to more than four hundred pediatricians attending the National Institute of Child Health Child Division meeting. He asked me for my slides from a paper I had just published on how to write a successful grant proposal in fewer than twenty pages that would be paid by the NIH. He used my slides to prepare his speech. As luck would have it, it snowed in Washington, D.C., that day, and those who live in Washington know that the government closes when there are flurries. He had to go pick up his wife after he spoke. I stayed at the meeting until the end. There were many questions stemming from his presentation, and he wasn't there to answer. The moderator asked for help, and I was able to answer every one of them since most of the questions stemmed from materials in my slides and paper. After I had answered the audience's questions, the Chief of Pediatrics came over to me and said, "I never knew you were a doctor." I said, "Is that important?" He said, "Well, I'm looking for a Deputy Director for the institute." I replied, "Well, that's perfect, because I have here my boss's curriculum vitae, and I want to give it to you." He said, "I'm not interested in him. I am interested in you."

My interview for the Deputy Director of the Child Health Institute was very different from what I had experienced before. Dr. Alexander knew my CV, my degrees, and my awards. He spent the interview time getting to know me. So the interview consisted of my human endeavors and performance in society. How do you treat patients? To what societies do you belong? How do you spend your time? And questions along that vein. After the interview, he assured me that as soon as he became the Director of the Institute (he had been performing in an acting capacity) that I would be his deputy. I left his office very happy, acting dignified. I thanked him.

It was about six p.m., and the corridors of the NIH were empty. I looked both ways, and then I shouted, screamed with joy, and threw all my papers in the air—and for a moment I felt just like Mary Tyler Moore!

I became the Deputy Director of the National Institute for Child Health, a position in which I served for almost four years. When things don't go your way, just know that there is a greater opportunity out there. Just have patience, lateralize if needed, and then get going. Don't lateralize to disappear but rather to build and grow—away from those who do not wish you well.

In October of 1998, the Cosmos Club in Washington, D.C., dropped its one-hundred-year-old men-only membership rule and admitted its first class of women (only 14 of the 771 members voted against). I was part of that first group of approximately forty women members. Since my husband was a member, I had heard that women could not go to the library or walk on the library's rug, read the books, or even go to the second floor where all these treasures were kept. Now that I was a member, my first visit was to the second-floor library. I walked and danced on the rug, read and touched the books. As an early feminist? As an avenger of women's rights? I don't really know, but it certainly made me feel good. Sometime thereafter, I dropped my membership.

> "When things don't go your way, just know that there is a greater opportunity out there. Just have patience, lateralize if needed, and then get going."

* * *

I do believe Joe continued his philandering during those years, but I never really knew—had no way to know. I was too busy working at the NIH and then being Surgeon General. In addition, he was never absent from his duties. He was always home at night. We didn't miss a single vacation together. Or maybe I refused to deal with the infidelities again so we both limped through the marriage until the divorce came in August 1994, although it wasn't finalized until after the house sold in 1998. Throughout our marriage, I felt he had been the best provider but not the best husband. When I would get angry at him, that is what I would tell him, as often as I could.

Part II

After overcoming a young life of challenges, I found myself at the pinnacle of public service. What follows are a series of stories and reflections that highlight the sheer pleasure of serving the public in a variety of capacities, while also recognizing that, even though one might reach a pinnacle, challenges lurk around every bend. It is in continuing to overcome these challenges that lessons are learned.

CHAPTER 6

The Pediatrician of the Nation

I have no idea why I was selected to be Surgeon General—the first woman and the first Hispanic in the office. I had no political power, no donations, and nothing to talk about regarding the members of the powerful Republican Eagles Club, the top donors to the Republican Party. But somehow, I got the job. It must have been the work I did when I didn't know others were watching, including Dr. James Mason (Director of the Centers for Disease Control [CDC]), Senator Hatch, and Dr. Louis Sullivan (Secretary of Health and Human Services).

In August of 1989 I got a call from Dr. Mason, the Assistant Secretary of Health (ASH), that would again change my life. Not surprisingly, I thought I had done something wrong, and he was calling to tell me so. Instead, he told me that Dr. Sullivan wanted to see me after Labor Day. I asked why. He didn't answer my question but asked me if there was ever a job in government that I wanted, what would that be? And I told him that I would like to be his deputy; he said that one was taken. And I said, "That's why I want it—because it is already taken, and I don't want to leave my deputy job at NIH."

After that phone conversation, I became suspicious and thought more about his request. I remembered that the Health Resources and Services Administration was currently without a Director. Although no woman had up to that point served as the Director of any of the agencies in the federal government, I decided that perhaps I was being considered for that position, and that was why Dr. Sullivan wanted to see me. I prepared as best I could by reading everything

I could find on HRSA. But I had also decided that I would tell him "no, thanks." I believed it was best to always leave them wanting.

I reported to HHS the day after Labor Day as requested to meet with Dr. Sullivan. I did not expect, ever in my life, the offer to become the United States Surgeon General. This was the first thing out of Dr. Sullivan's mouth. I screamed—his head fell back—he asked, surprised, had I not heard about it before coming? I said, "No." And he proceeded to tell me what he would like to see in the candidate. I readily accepted his offer.

After this, his Chief of Staff walked in and asked if everything was okay. Dr. Sullivan said, "Yes. She has accepted the offer." And then this Chief of Staff asked me what had I done for the Republican Party. I said, "Nothing." He looked at Dr. Sullivan with disbelief, almost implying, "You interviewed her, and she cannot serve." I told him that since I was a career public health officer, The Hatch Act prohibited me from participating in politics. That saved the day. The rest of the formalities included meeting with the office of personnel at the White House and President Bush's Chief of Staff, which went off without a hitch.

When I found out, I was honored and panicked at the same time. First, because unlike many others who had served as US Surgeons General before me, I was neither in academia nor in private industry. Second, I would be succeeding Dr. C. Everett Koop, who had become a legend in his own time. Dr. Koop had raised the visibility of the office of Surgeon General thanks in part to his quit smoking initiatives and his stature and leadership during the AIDS epidemic. He had served for two terms—eight years. Who could follow in his footsteps? My insecurities were exacerbated during the delay between my nomination (November 1, 1989) and my swearing in (March 1990). My mind was full of worries. What are my responsibilities? Do I respond to the President? Or to the Secretary of HHS? Or to the ASH? During that time, I was sent to Geneva so I would be out of the country during the FBI clearance part of the vetting process. When I came back from Geneva, I was briefed at the Department of HHS. Then, the congressional hearings occurred. The day after, when I was driving on Constitution Avenue in Washington, D.C., I heard on the radio that I had been confirmed as US Surgeon General. Although in one hundred years, five US Surgeons General have been both Surgeon General and ASH, I would not be one of them.

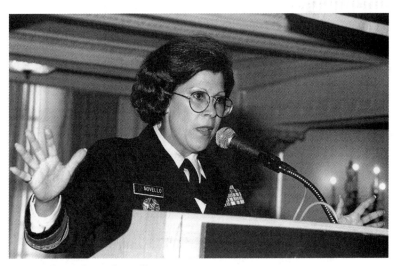

Dr. Novello speaks emphatically.

Usually, the swearing in of the Surgeon General takes place on the seventh floor of HHS—200 Pennsylvania Avenue. When I met the Inspector General of HHS, he said, "Where are you going to be sworn in?" And I replied, "If I make it, right here." And he said, "Oh no you're not. You're the first woman Surgeon General ever. You have to be sworn in at the White House. And the person who will swear you in will be the first female Justice on the US Supreme Court." I said, "You've got to be kidding." He said, "No." And sure enough, that was what happened.

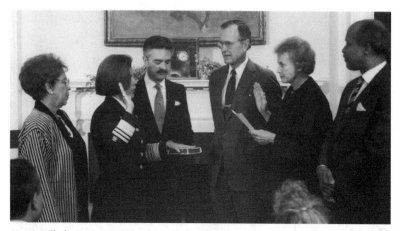

Dr. Novello being sworn in as the 14th US Surgeon General by Justice Sandra Day O'Connor in the Roosevelt Room at the White House. Left to right: Dr. Novello's mother, Ana Delia Flores; Dr. Antonia Novello; her husband, Dr. Joseph Novello; President George H. W. Bush; Justice Sandra Day O'Connor; and Dr. Louis Sullivan, Secretary of the Department of Health and Human Services.

There had never been a female Vice Admiral (three star) in the armed forces or in the uniformed services. I was making a huge leap from Captain (my rank in the PHS) to Vice Admiral (the rank of Surgeon General). Dr. Koop donated his epaulettes with the rank to me. Unfortunately, I looked like a South American dictator with my small shoulders and those huge epaulettes! The first three-star epaulettes for a woman were made just for me.

As had been predicted, my swearing in as US Surgeon General took place at the Roosevelt Room in the White House on March 9, 1990. Supreme Court Justice Sandra Day O'Connor swore me in with President George H. W. Bush, Dr. Sullivan, Dr. Mason, Senator Hatch, Representative Silvio Conte of Massachusetts, my mother, my husband, his parents, my nieces, and many dear friends present. My remarks included that my motto as Surgeon General would be "good science and good sense." After the swearing in, I was approached by one of the President's assistants who said the President wanted to see me in the Oval Office, and that I could bring people with me. I brought Mami, Joe, and my three nieces.

Afterward, there was a reception. I was so happy but lonely and somewhat afraid of the task ahead. From the White House, we went to the airport and flew to Denver, Colorado. I had been invited to be on stage with John Denver there. I had promised my Director

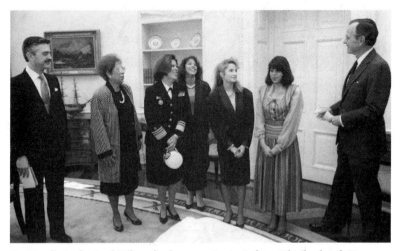

Dr. Novello in the Oval Office after her swearing in. Left to right: *husband, Dr. Joseph Novello; mother, Ana Delia Flores; Dr. Antonia Novello; niece, Mayra Coello; Joe's niece, Holly Weirsma; niece, Tanya Coello; and President George H. W. Bush.*

at Child Health that I would do this for him months before I was confirmed, so I kept my word. We had a connecting flight to Denver and as we were sitting in the airport, there was a news story on the television about the swearing in of the new Surgeon General—me. That was when I realized that it was true. Me, this little girl from Fajardo. John Denver introduced me to the audience, and I gave a little speech. Then it was back to Washington, D.C., to start the job and my new life.

One of the things that terrified me was that I would be following Dr. Koop. Not only was he an extremely well-respected leader and physician but as a true public health officer, not a political appointee; he had also been my boss. And he was perceived as a god in public health. I couldn't have bigger, larger footsteps to follow than his. He had served so many years and had become bigger than history. He served as Surgeon General during both of President Ronald Reagan's terms.

When Dr. Koop was my boss, he nominated me to serve as the Chair of his Revitalization of the Public Health Service task force. I had very close contact with Dr. Koop for that entire year. There was a team of four, and I would take portions of the final report as they were drafted to him for his review. He was pleased with our results. As part of that effort, we established a policy for what a flag holder's tenure should be. In the Public Health Service, flag holders or flag officers (officers of a minimum certain rank have the right to fly a flag) will hold one of the following ranks: Rear Admiral lower half or upper half (one and two stars, respectively), Vice Admiral (three stars), or Admiral (four stars). Flag officers get more money and also can serve more years before retirement. For every star, you can remain three years past retirement after twenty years of service. But you cannot practice your specialty once you are a flag officer.

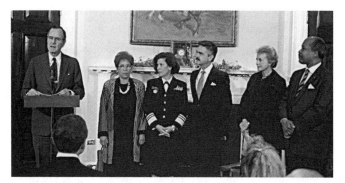

President George H. W. Bush speaks during Dr. Antonia Novello's swearing in. Left to right: mother, Ana Delia Flores; Dr. Antonia Novello; husband, Dr. Joseph Novello; Justice Sandra Day O'Connor; and Secretary of Health and Human Services, Dr. Louis Sullivan.

The Public Health Service had only one four star—an Admiral who is the ASH. There is one Vice Admiral, the Surgeon General, with three stars. And there were about twenty-eight flag officers scattered around various agencies out of total personnel of about seventy-five hundred. Once people get a star, that star stays with them until they die, retire, or leave the Public Health Service. There were cases in which I was requested to give flags that I thought were inappropriate, and I didn't. In other cases, I gave flags to people at the NIH and at the CDC who never expected to make flag officer during their career, although such were well deserved. I also gave one flag to the Indian Health Service. In addition, I created regulations to give two flags, not necessarily approved by the Revitalization Task Force but that I thought were very important for the Public Health Service. They were for those who did important jobs but would never oversee a health agency—one for the Chief of Personnel and one for the Surgeon General's Chief of Staff. Their jobs deserved such recognition.

The life of the Surgeon General is full of invitations, hearings, meetings, and reports, so you really have to have some stamina to last through hours over which you have no control. Even if you get to the office before eight a.m., you will be lucky to get home at nine thirty p.m. And even then, you have to prepare for the next day when you might open a center, requiring travel to another state and then an immediate return as you have something the morning after. At first, I was overwhelmed. How do I tell my husband that he is going to see me so infrequently? And I do take responsibility—I put these responsibilities on myself, which I think makes it more difficult. I have always been extremely demanding of and hard on myself. I still had all of the home responsibilities as well: ensuring that the house was supplied and cooking dinner for Joe every night. He didn't care how late we ate as long as we had dinner together, sitting at the table.

Every day was like a ping-pong game or tennis. They were throwing balls constantly—for news—and I had to make sure that I hit them back from my side of the tennis court. It had to be the truth and it had to be backed up by health and science. There were pitfalls everywhere.

* * *

My first lesson as Surgeon General was to not invent policy out of fear. It is very ego-boosting to be in front of the microphone, but you must relinquish it before you do anything you will regret later. So I learned that just because you have the microphone, time, and attention, it is not appropriate to invent policy just to keep the attention of the press. I also learned that if you do not know the answer, say you do not know but find the answer immediately and have it delivered to the person who made the request. Never make something up. If you do, you will destroy your credibility.

I saw my position as Surgeon General almost as being a member of an academic university. I had known Dr. Mason when he was the head of the CDC, and I had known Dr. Sullivan when he was a member of the board of the Cancer Institute at the NIH. I viewed the arrangement almost as if I were the Dean, Dr. Sullivan was the President, and Dr. Mason was the Chancellor. I took care of them in their roles as I would have had I been the Dean.

I also realized that I needed to create an agenda for my four years as Surgeon General. The agenda was important since there was so little money allocated to the office—just enough for salaries, travel, and minimal expenses. You had to invent what you didn't have and most of the other agencies would send you a special assistant—which came without cost in dollars and cents. The cost, however, was that the other agency then got to dictate areas of emphasis to advance their own agendas. My agenda included tobacco, women's health issues, vaccinations, underage drinking, and AIDS. And whereas Dr. Koop could dictate, I needed to be diplomatic while working on the agenda.

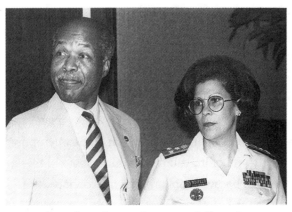

Dr. Novello in dress whites with Dr. Louis Sullivan, Secretary of the Department of Health and Human Services.

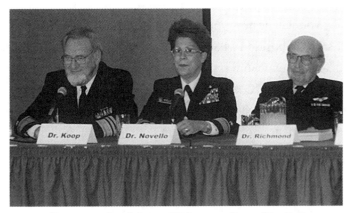

Dr. Novello on a panel with former US Surgeons General Dr. C. Everett Koop and Dr. Julius Richmond.

As the first woman Surgeon General and the first Hispanic, I think too many people placed too many hopes on my shoulders. They forgot or did not understand what my job was all about. They wanted me to be the Hispanic Surgeon General to service the Hispanic community. I told them that I work for all the people—not just a group or a race. And I served at the pleasure of the President approved by the US Congress. Still, I knew and felt that I would be a role model

instantaneously, and I took that very seriously. Especially because
I knew that for Hispanics honor is more important than life. And I
was not about to bring dishonor to any of them in anything that
I did. I just could not fail.

I also learned about the politics of the job. Your speechwriter,
your Public Affairs Officer, and your Chief of Staff are all in the job
because they have excelled in politics outside of the office of the Surgeon General. I learned to write my own speeches. I learned when
to go through them and when to go around them in order to accomplish what I wanted to accomplish as Surgeon General.

As Surgeon General I learned that you don't just give the audience a lot of data, you must leave them with solutions. I had impact
communicating because I was the Surgeon General, but that was not
enough. I had to give people something at the end—a plan of action.
I learned not to leave the audience with a problem and not tell them
what to do.

Another lesson was that half of the people came to listen to what
I had to say, and half wanted to see if I was wrong. So when I told
them a number such as a percentage or the number of cases of a
disease, I was as factual as possible for the moment and time. I was
obsessed with my credibility.

I did not want to do my first press conference in Washington,
D.C. I wanted it to be in Puerto Rico, and it was. My hometown
school band was at the airport very proudly playing music in my
honor. Mami and I got off the plane together. They took us in a
caravan to my hometown, and the baseball arena was packed with
students from all the classes from juniors to seniors, and they were
excited. I was crying. So was Mami. It was an intense scene. I spoke
to the group with encouraging words telling them if I could make
it, so could they. It was a great experience for Mami, too. This was
her daughter who used to be one of the children on those bleachers.
From there, Mami and I were escorted to the Caribe Hilton where

we had been given a beautiful suite of rooms to stay in, to continue my visit on the island.

Every time there was a knock on the door, another beautiful arrangement of flowers was delivered. It looked like an English garden in my room. I was surrounded by flowers. Eventually I requested that those flowers be distributed to all the nursing homes in the capital area as well as local cemeteries. Who knows, some of those flowers might have ended up on the graves of the unknown, the poor, or the forgotten—courtesy of one of their own—but this time from the woman in uniform.

And then it was time to get ready for the evening at the Casino of Puerto Rico. A formal dress. Immaculate hair. In the old Casino of Puerto Rico there was a huge stairway, conjoined at the bottom and then splitting partway up with one stairway going up on the left and the other on the right. At the top was the reception area. I was almost at the top of the stairway when one of my shoes came off. It went all the way down this huge stairway. I had felt like a princess going up those stairs—really like Cinderella. I was holding the rail and the shoe falling off reminded me that I was human and not perfect. With the beautiful dress and the perfect makeup—I probably looked quite regal. And all of a sudden, I lost my shoe!

Waiting for me at the entrance to the reception area were the President of the university, the Secretary of State, the entire list of who's who. We were going to have a receiving line. And they were all watching the shoe go down and down the stairs. Almost in slow motion. And I am guessing that my mouth was wide open. The job made me big, but I was still the little girl from Fajardo and the Prince was not there to put the shoe back on. Joe had stayed at home; our marriage was in trouble. Instead, I had traveled with my mother and my nieces. But someone brought the shoe back and I was me again.

Back on the mainland after the press conference, my first speech as Surgeon General in D.C. was at a high school football game, and

I was supposed to talk about tobacco. What a topic! What a terrible first encounter with members of the public. The people attending the football game wanted to hear go, go, go! Fight, fight, fight! And I was talking about Don't do this and Don't do that. My speechwriter and my press person said that my speech and I were the worst in the world. They didn't take any ownership for their part of the scheduling or writing. I kept quiet, but I knew it was time to say good-bye to the press person. The final straw was when an Italian group invited me to speak, and she told them, "She is too busy, contact her later." Needless to say, I never heard from them again, and my press person and my speechwriter were gone voluntarily within a few months of my being in office.

Because my confidence in my speaking was severely impacted by my performance at the football game, by the time of my second speech, I sat on the toilet and cried. I had to learn that my survival was in my hands. I must address the problems of the country, without forgetting to mention the President, and be sure that my political assistants did not derail whatever I was trying to say. Foremost, I must never lose the public trust. All of that was on my mind. What was the best for me and how could I best meet the public health needs of the country?

Fortunately for me, shortly after that second speech, Joe walked into the bathroom when I was getting ready one morning and said, "Please remember that you only have one boss. You only obey one God and one President. And the latter will not object to the former. So do what you have to do. Until you are savvier and can discern who is who, the American public—for which you were selected to serve—remains your biggest advocate or your biggest blocker. Provide them with facts and transparency while using diplomacy. They will in turn become your most trusted ally and you will succeed. Just give yourself time. God did not create everything in one day."

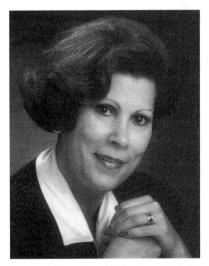

Portrait of Dr. Antonia Novello as 14th US Surgeon General.

I never dreamed that one of my responsibilities as US Surgeon General would be furnishing my office. Because of the small budget allocated to the office, I needed to get furniture. I heard about a room full of furniture at the White House—left over from the previous administrations—and I got what I needed. I still had to buy the furniture but at a lower price. I painted the steel-gray desks in black and bought fabric to reupholster instead of buying new sofas and chairs. It took a while for my furniture to be reupholstered. Then I realized why. Within the federal government, the job of reupholstering furniture goes to the prison system. The prisoners thought the client was the *Attorney* General; not understanding it was for the *Surgeon* General, and they did everything they could to delay the order.

When the reupholstered furniture did arrive, I chose not to use cushions to decorate. Instead, I used Cabbage Patch dolls on the gray sofa at the entrance to my office. Each doll had a disability. One was blind. One was deaf. One was

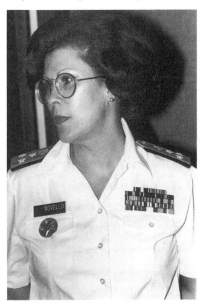

Dr. Novello in dress whites.

otherwise physically disabled. And so forth. These dolls allowed me to observe the behavior of my guests from behind the comfort of my desk. Some sat on top of them. Some threw them on the floor. Others did their best to hold the dolls until they were called to see me.

This maneuver allowed me to understand my visitors at least superficially—who was a decent human being or not—before they were in my office in front of me. It turned out that I was wrong very few times. It was an eye opener for me as to how people treat objects that depict pain for some families and then nonchalantly come into my view like angels asking for favors. I was able to know them through their behavior—knowing what to expect and how far I could help. As I believe so strongly, "compassion" for others is not a dirty word.

At the time I was Surgeon General, AIDS was a very big issue. Dr. Koop had written the first report on AIDS, and the second report came out during my tenure. During my tenure, treatments were starting to become available and huge sensitivity was required. Before, people were dying of pneumonia, and nobody wanted to say they were HIV positive. There was a huge stigma. There was also national guilt because people had not been taken care of appropriately as it had been deemed in many people's eyes a "gay disease." We needed to acknowledge that the people who were getting sick were Americans and human beings who needed care. They deserved treatment. They deserved care. They deserved respect. And they deserved not to be stigmatized.

One of the issues early in the AIDS epidemic was that quite a few active military personnel became HIV positive at a time of both great stigma toward people with the disease and a lack of available treatments. We at the Public Health Service were asked about the possibility of taking them on as part of our workforce. Dr. Mason came and asked for my opinion. I talked about the US Public Health service being a movable force—people were constantly assigned to locations based on need and could be transferred with very little notice. Thus, it would look awkward to have all these personnel at jobs that were probably desk assignments. I felt that in the quest to help, we could indirectly be violating their right to privacy, causing their peers to question why they were not part of the movable team and questioning if something was wrong with them. I think Dr. Mason understood, and we both decided above all to protect these individuals' privacy. They already had suffered enough. They needed care and empathy, not additional judgment. So the military continued to keep them under their care.

As Surgeon General, my office got the first call made to the federal government from Magic Johnson when he tested positive for and developed AIDS. What a man of character and ability to think about how he might be able to help others through his story! I also immediately got a call from the Press Director for the Secretary of HHS telling me that any new call from Magic Johnson was to be directed immediately to her office, not to mine. Apparently, the grapevine in HHS was quite active, reinforcing what I had suspected all along—that there were no secrets in government. That Press Director was heard to say that if I did not obey the directive, she would "hang me by my tits." She did not tell me directly, however. They did not invite me to the HHS AIDS monthly committee meeting, of which I was a member, when Magic Johnson attended. I showed up to the meeting, anyway, because the grapevine was working overtime, and I was told about it. I thanked Magic Johnson for his courage, grabbed a chair, stood on top of it (to be close to his height), and had my picture taken with him. I know that was a clear demonstration of chutzpah—to show up those who treated me like I was invisible when they didn't want to share the limelight with the Surgeon General even though AIDS was under my jurisdiction.

During the AIDS crisis, groups like ACT UP would come into offices including the NIH (Dr. Anthony Fauci's office), the Federal

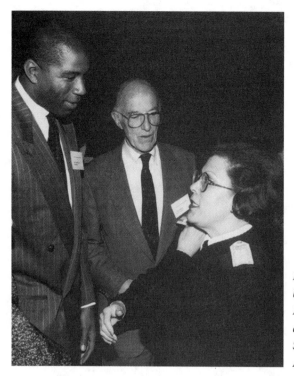

Dr. Novello with basketball great Magic Johnson during a Health and Human Services monthly AIDS meeting.

Drug Administration (FDA), and the office of the US Surgeon General to create a newsworthy spectacle. When my turn came, a small but very vociferous group came to my office to talk, or fight, or just learn about what we were doing for the cause. I remember that as the main spokesperson was about to be heard, he glanced at the largest wall of my office where a piece of the AIDS quilt[1] was hanging. To my amazement, he got very quiet, and then he started to cry. In empathy, I started to cry as well. The person acknowledged on the quilt had been his partner, and here was the Office of the Surgeon General honoring his memory. It was a beautiful and silent moment of mutual understanding and respect, establishing that prejudice or stigmatization had no place in my life or in my office. Since that day

---

[1]The AIDS Memorial Quilt, begun in 1985, has fifty thousand panels honoring people who died during the AIDS epidemic.

I have felt that the gay community understood where I stood regarding their cause. I have never had any problems helping them and/or listening to their needs whether at HHS as Surgeon General or as Commissioner of Health in New York State.

Around this same time, a report was made on national television that women were not contracting AIDS. This was obviously not true, and I had to deal with the reports and the reporter. The station eventually retracted that story. Women were contracting AIDS through sex, so we had to protect all women, including pregnant women, breastfeeding women, and their infants. It took time, but we succeeded.

In addition to AIDS, I decided that one of the planks of my agenda would be medical care for the Hispanic population. No one had ever taken up that mantle before, and I believed that addressing Hispanic health was crucial. I divided the country into five areas and selected five points, ranging from prevention to research, that needed to be addressed for each area. At that time, the CDC did not break out Hispanics as a race—they grouped Hispanics into "others," so I felt discussing a Hispanic agenda was crucial at the time. We needed to be more than "others." Sadly, the same agenda that my group worked and reported on is still in place today. Similarly, not all the agenda points from research to implementation to prevention have yet been fully addressed by the government, and every year I see the agenda report changing just the name of the Secretary and the date—but the needs remain the same.

There was a time when requests would come in for speaking engagements for the Surgeon General more than for the Assistant Secretary of Health or the Secretary of Health and Human Services. As Surgeon General, I could talk about illness, disease, cures, the latest in science—things like that. The ASH or the Secretary of HHS, however, spoke more about appropriations and money so their requests to speak were more limited.

I got a call from the White House one day saying that I had not mentioned the name of the President in a recent speech. I asked which speech, and the woman said the one I had given the day before. That day I had given a speech on AIDS, and I really could not mention the name of the President since I was talking about funding and caring about the individuals who had contracted the disease. This topic was something that the group to which I was speaking felt not enough was being done, and what was being done was not being done well. Thus, I explained that I had tried to avoid making negative press for the President by mentioning his name in my speech. The White House let this one go, but it made me understand that I was being watched like a hawk.

The second dealing I had with the HHS Secretary's Press Director was quite different from the one concerning Magic Johnson. A young girl had sustained permanent brain damage and was permanently incapacitated after teenagers drunk on Cisco (a fortified wine cooler drink), called "liquid crack" on the streets, threw rocks and Cisco bottles from an overpass onto her car. I called all the presidents of the liquor, champagne, wine, and beer companies in the US to talk about the incident. I told them that the wine and spirits industry was being damaged by underage drinking, and I told them as well that situations like this prompted adherence to regulations or else. I told the attendees that this was a meeting among us—there was to be no press coverage, and if they broke that request, then I would follow with my own press conference.

At this meeting, unbeknownst to me, was Mr. Gallo, the biggest winemaker at the time. He told everyone attending that I had clout: "Listen to her," he said, "she has the power to shut us down. I know, I was there during prohibition." Then he left the room. I swear I heard the music from *The Godfather* as he walked out—with his red carnation in the lapel of his pinstriped suit.

The Press Director sent me a note after the meeting calling me a "10"—unbelievable. Maybe it was because I had learned how to manage my job and my responsibilities in the office. Or maybe it was because I acted and talked to all those men at the meeting as one CEO to another.

No notes were taken at the meeting. We agreed on what actions to pursue on our word of honor. Three months later, I was able to move Cisco where it belonged—behind the counter as an alcoholic drink in a dark bottle, not in the refrigerated area as a wine cooler, in pink.

Many years later, as Health Commissioner of the State of New York, I was invited to a dinner, and the president of Cisco was there sitting across from me. It was very awkward. I wasn't sure if he had tied both jobs to the same woman—but it was very difficult for me to swallow my food once I knew who was paying for the dinner.

Before I became Surgeon General, the tobacco companies had written a memo stating that I should be selected because I had never said anything that would cause problems for them. I am sure they would have liked that memo to disappear—because I did see it. Not only did I take on Old Joe Camel—a caricature used by the cigarette companies to market to the young—but I also realized that the cost of a package of cigarettes needed to increase. Every time the price of a package increased, the smoking rate decreased. The tobacco companies did not expect that from me, nor did they expect my opposition to Old Joe Camel.

I was walking down Michigan Avenue in Chicago during the American Medical Association yearly meeting accompanied by the Surgeons General of the Army, Navy, and Air Force. We were all marching against Old Joe Camel. As I was stepping out on Michigan Avenue, I got a call from the White House stating that I could not mention Old Joe Camel. I was flabbergasted. Someone important in the presidential circle had ties to the tobacco industry and was using their clout. The protest against Old Joe Camel was not new; for me, it was a personal battle against Old Joe and the selling of cigarettes to youth. I asked the person who called how I could protest Old Joe if I couldn't mention him by name. So I asked if I would be able to point at the camel instead. I guess they were amused—and said yes. Little did they know that I had a huge poster of Old Joe that I was carrying while I was marching along Michigan Avenue. I kept pointing to his face with my finger down. An award for the best poster against Old Joe was given at that time. Success. The point was made. Remember, necessity is the mother of invention.

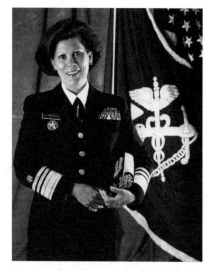

Portrait of Dr. Antonia Novello as 14th US Surgeon General with the medical flag in the background.

At one point, I was asked to speak at Barnard College where the students opposed my stance on abortion. I believed, like many others at the time, that abortion should only be performed when the health of the woman was in danger. As I started my speech, many young women pulled out hangers and held them high in protest. I knew the speech contained important information for them, and I proceeded to give it. I thought, the devil knows more by being old than by being the devil, and it is going to be difficult for them to keep those hangers up for an hour. As I spoke, time passed, and the hangers came down. Finally, they applauded my speech. They had their opinions and I had mine. But I was older and with knowledge at hand, diplomacy, and respect. Especially since

> "Remember, necessity is the mother of invention."

I had not given an in-your-face speech, we as people were able to succeed in civility and mutual respect. They respected me, and I in turn respected them.

One of the most coveted invitations in Washington while I was Surgeon General was to celebrate Queen Elizabeth's visit to the US in 1991. I was seated at the table with President George H. W. Bush. He was to my left. To his left was Queen Elizabeth II. She had two ladies-in-waiting with her. Joe was seated at the next table over with Prince Philip. The Queen was dressed in a beautiful gown wearing a diamond necklace, earrings, and a tiara. In addition, she had many medals with ribbons as did her ladies-in-waiting. She ate very little, mostly moving the food around her plate with her fork. The protocol was such that I could not address the Queen. She spoke mostly with her ladies-in-waiting and with the President. But what an honor it was for me to be seated at that table.

Barbara Bush, the President's wife, convened what she called her "kitchen cabinet." These were meetings where women agency heads would meet with Mrs. Bush at the White House and discuss the issues of the land. She would listen, and I believe that she communicated some of the issues that were discussed with the President. I was very thankful that I could communicate concerns from the HIV-positive community to her.

I was invited to many dinners at the White House during my tenure as Surgeon General. One evening, Mrs. Bush had put a purse on the table that looked just like Millie, her dog. Millie was ill, but here was a little white purse that looked just like her. I said, "Mrs. Bush, that is a wonderful, wonderful purse." And she said, "Yes, it was given to me by Judith Leiber." And I said, "Wow. It is something else. Before I die, I'm going to get myself a Judith Leiber purse." And she looked at me and said, "Really?" And I said, "Yes." The woman sitting next to Mrs. Bush was Judith Leiber: a regal woman with white hair in a black dress. A week later, I got a Judith Leiber purse in the mail—a very small black cocktail purse that I still have. I use it often and I never put it on the table because it would disappear; such purses are coveted, valuable items. Some of them I have seen

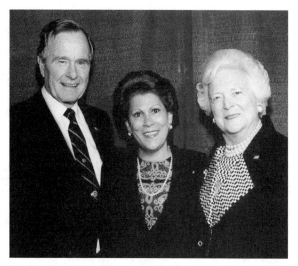

Dr. Novello with President George H. W. Bush and Barbara Bush.

displayed as objects of art in china cabinets in homes around the country. I am glad my purse was a very small one.

UNICEF had a new children's agenda, and the United Nations had decided to make that a reality. There were ten items on the agenda for infancy protection that included vaccination for all children, breast-feeding, and adding iodine to the salt of the world. President Bush and all the big honchos in Washington came to hear a presentation by the UNICEF Director Mr. James P. Grant at the Hall of the UN in 1990. For some reason, we all went to church—an Episcopalian service. Attending the service was Margaret Thatcher, then Prime Minister of England. I was sitting two rows behind Dr. Sullivan, the Secretary of HHS, when I heard President Bush say, "Margaret, come I want you to meet somebody." And the Secretary of HHS, who was in front of me, stood up, but the President bypassed him and motioned for Margaret Thatcher to meet me. The President said, "This is the Surgeon General of the United States, a woman." I was about to faint. She said, "How are you?" and made small talk with me. She had her purse on her side. Her hair was perfect. The dress—impeccable.

Wow! I was in heaven. I was so elated at having had the opportunity to be introduced to such an important woman but also quite concerned because the President had bypassed the Secretary and had come my way instead. I kept a very low profile after that morning.

I'll never forget this: I was getting ready to do a press conference, but I am a woman first, and I wanted to do my nails. At the time, I was wearing red fingernail polish. As I was doing my nails, the whole

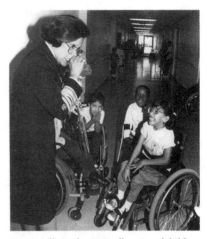

Dr. Novello makes a small group of children laugh as she tells them she isn't going to get into a wheelchair and race them. Photo courtesy of Society of Education and Rehabilitation of Puerto Rico (SER de PR).

bottle of nail polish fell on my lap. My press conference was in one hour, and there was no way I could have my skirt dry cleaned in that small amount of time. Oh, my God, what was I going to do?

I went to see Dr. Mason, the ASH, who was a serious and very important member of the Mormon church. I went in and I said, "Dr. Mason, can I borrow your pants?" I thought I was going to be ousted from the Public Health Service. He looked at me and said, "You want to what?" And I said, "Could I please have a pair of pants?" He said, "What do you need them for?" And I moved my hand and showed him the massive red fingernail polish stain on the front of my skirt. He looked at me in disbelief and said, "They are in the closet." So I went to the closet and got a pair of pants. They were almost a foot longer than they should have been on me—over my shoes. I wore my uniform from the top and Dr. Mason's pants from the bottom, and I gave the press conference sitting behind my desk. It went well.

No one in the press corps would ever know that I was wearing his pants. But that was the talk of the department for about a month. We would laugh because at that time Dr. Mason was still not an Admiral. He was one rank under my own rank. He was a two star, and I was a three star. I never let him forget that in his office at least once—I wore the pants.

I became a member of the American Academy of Achievement during my tenure as Surgeon General. At one of the meetings, I was holding my glasses in my hand. Somebody came up from the rear and hugged me so hard that I crushed my glasses. I was about to protest, but I turned around to see who that person was. It was Tom Selleck. He proceeded to apologize and wanted to buy me new ones. I did not accept, but I still remember the bear hug.

That was one memorable meeting. Another memorable meeting of the organization stemmed from a letter I had received during my term as Surgeon General from a six- or seven-year-old African American girl. She said, "My name is Antonia. And my intention is to be the Surgeon General of the United States. Make sure you do good. Don't ruin my name." Many years later, the American Academy of Achievement's meeting was in the state where she lived. Here came this young woman who looked at me and said, "You were the Surgeon General?" I said, "Yes." She said, "I am Antonia. I was the one who wrote you that letter. And now I am like you at the University of Michigan in medical school. Thank you so much for making it possible for me to come to meet you." And then I invited her to sit at my table next to Colin Powell. She made me proud of what she had become, and hopefully one day I can give her my epaulettes—you just never know! But this time, they will be the right size.

Dr. Mason had a driver and so did I. But one day, his driver was absent, and Dr. Mason had to get to Dulles Airport. Unbeknownst to me—and because he was my boss in need—he took my driver and left for the airport.

I didn't have time to tell him that my driver had just arrived from Puerto Rico. He knew how to drive, but he didn't know Washington, D.C., or the English alphabet and therefore he kept looking for letters in the Spanish alphabet like double "l" or "ñ." Unfortunately, Dr. Mason missed his plane twice—once at Dulles Airport and once at National Airport.

He was fuming when he arrived back at the office. I was aware that he had a terrible temper and was trying to save everyone from his anger. I put on a hat and jacket, saluted him, and said, "I am ready to drive you, sir." The tension was palpable. He burst out laughing at my attire, and I felt that from that moment on he would ask first to use anybody else's driver—especially if they had just arrived in the capital and spoke no English.

I was having a meeting with a man in my office in the evening, maybe five thirty or six o'clock. My back was to the window of my office and my guest was in front of me. Five or six minutes into the conversation, he was putting his finger up and kind of pointing. I

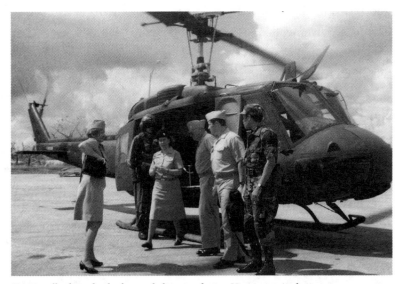

Dr. Novello disembarks from a helicopter during Hurricane Andrew.

was thinking to myself that this man had Parkinson's or he had a problem. So I paid no attention. But he kept pointing, curving his finger, like something was behind me. Finally, I took the hint and looked— there was a mouse behind me. And, not surprisingly, I was not very nice. I screamed bloody murder and had forgotten that, unfortunately, my secretary would be more panicked than me. Now the mouse was on top of the desk, and we were both screaming for somebody to come and get this mouse.

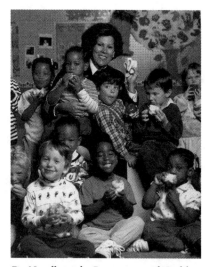

Dr. Novello at the Department of Health and Human Services day care center surrounded by children eating fruit. (The girl on the far right is the one trying to eat a wooden apple!)

Two people appeared about five minutes later in white uniforms to dispose of the mouse. I was very surprised that the US government had people in white uniforms that can get rid of mice and rats from government property. From then on, I always looked before I sat in that particular area!

During my time as Surgeon General, there was a day care center at the Department of HHS where employees could bring their children. We took a wonderful picture with the children in the place, giving fruit to those who sat up close. One little girl came in late and was at the back of the group, and we had no more apples. So we gave her a wooden apple. Her face is precious as she was trying to bite the apple. Since the time that we took the picture, at least two of the HHS Secretaries after me decided to take the same kind of picture. They didn't know that the little girl in the back was chewing on a wooden apple. And the resultant pictures are full copies of the original.

As Surgeon General, I made many trips to the Native American reservations of North and South Dakota—the Lakota Nation and the Blackfeet Nation. On one of my many visits, they invited me to dinner—not that day but the next day. When I asked why, they said it was because the meat had to be prepared. I didn't understand, so I asked again. To my amazement, I was shown the cans of groceries they were given for food supplements. They were all big and gray, and they only said "meat," "milk," "flour," "sugar," and so forth. Nothing like the food we buy in the grocery store with preparation directions or calorie and protein content.

I looked at the meat can—they opened it and according to the directions, the contents had to be dropped in water. To my surprise, the can was half meat and half pure grease and fat. It needed twenty-four hours so the fat could move to the top and be removed. When I looked at it, my heart bled. I recalled that, apart from alcoholism, the two major causes of death among Native Americans were heart disease and kidney disease. Under the guise of helping them by giving them food, we could be causing them long-term harm. Some Native Americans had to drive a hundred miles to a dialysis center. I wondered if the food the government was giving them was causing hypertension and diabetes and/or obesity.

I discussed this situation with Department of Agriculture personnel. They said it was free food, and they didn't mince their words when they said it was better than nothing. They seemed to think I was a busybody. What a grave disappointment for me. At that moment, I felt I wanted to become a lobbyist for the Native American people, regardless of what the Department of Agriculture personnel thought of me.

I was invited to a sacred ceremony of the Native Americans at the sweat lodges. A sweat lodge is a dark, intensely private and hot lodge where, after you enter, you are surrounded by others. The ambiance is very conducive for praying and for appreciating what God has given you, while coal burns in a pit. The only problem during my visit was that as a woman you have to be clean, meaning "not menstruating." Therefore, a Chief of the Lakotas asked me if I was menstruating. I thought I was going to die after the question. I was not menstruating, and I said so. To my amazement, as I said no and entered the lodge, drums started playing loudly and constantly. To this day, I wonder if the whole state of North Dakota learned that the Surgeon General of the United States was not menstruating. It was worth it, though, to be able to participate in the sweat lodge. It was a beautiful feeling of peace, prayer, and retrospection. I was so honored to have been invited and, more than anything, that I was not menstruating.

Whenever I visited one of the Native American nations, there always was a powwow. I had the privilege of going to the Pine Ridge Reservation in South Dakota and visiting Wounded Knee. I really did feel like I was on sacred ground. I got to fly over the Black Hills, which are sacred to the Sioux people. The Native American nations were extremely pleased to show and share the beauty of their land with me. During my years as Surgeon General, I helped the Sioux defeat the liquor company that was trying to sell alcoholic beverages with the name of "Crazy Horse." In a way, I became an advocate for the Native American nations, and we ended up respecting and loving each other.

One of my trips to the Dakotas tested all my diplomacy skills. I remember coming down from the Cessna in my dress whites into a warm and welcoming crowd waiting to receive me. As I looked into the crowd there was a boy in a wheelchair with what appeared to be cerebral palsy. He had flowers in his hand that he was to give to me. As he gave them to me, he inadvertently grabbed my breast with his other hand. I didn't know what to do, but I certainly heard a gasp. I am still not sure if that gasp came from me or from the crowd. I proceeded to place my hands on his face, rubbed his head, and slowly removed his hand while I took the flowers away from him. The day

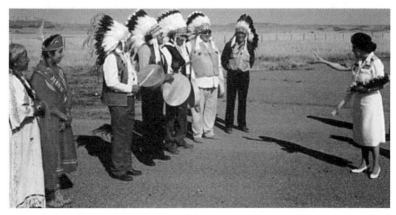

Dr. Novello holds a bouquet of flowers while meeting with a group of Native Americans.

was saved. My breast was fine—though my ego was bruised—but we did well. The boy was so happy that it was worth it. It made his day; he felt important.

I became very close to the Chief of the Pine Ridge reservation. He would frequently call my office whenever there was something he thought I could help with. His name was George Kicking Woman. I did work up the nerve to ask him how he got his name—was it a family name or a tradition? He laughed so hard but never said a word regarding the reason for his name, nor did he answer my question. I hope I didn't offend him. Between his name and that of his assistant, I had a lot to learn. His assistant's name was The One That Leaves at Night." My assistant said she knew a few of those and the conversation ended.

During my tenure as Surgeon General, the variety of things I engaged in was seemingly endless. For example, in addition to moving Cisco behind the counter, at my urging and with significant effort on my part, seven reports were produced on underage drinking. Because they were paid for by the Inspector General of the Department of HHS, they were published by that department and the Inspector General's name (Kusserow) appears printed on the title page. They were really Surgeon General reports, though. A compilation of all seven reports was made and the resulting booklet distributed to all high schools in the US. Someday I would like those books to be given under the name of the Office of the Surgeon General.

Sometimes you have to do what you have to do. Duty calls. I was invited to the training ship of the US Coast Guard, and I had to go. We at Public Health are the medical doctors for the Coast Guard, so as Surgeon General I was invited for a ride on the Coast Guard training ship.

The ocean was so rough where the Coast Guard ship was anchored that they dropped me from a helicopter down to the deck, and I came down using the rope ladder. There were two rows of men—one on each side—and I walked through the middle as they were welcoming me on board. I went like a drunk from one side of men to the other while someone kept blowing a whistle for the welcoming ceremony.

I noticed that my host was wearing two anti-seasickness patches—one behind each of her ears. She was wearing my patch, so I did not get one. That was not a good omen.

I passed through the kitchen and the smell of mushroom soup was so pungent that I wanted to vomit, and I did. I was taken to my quarters. As I tried to lie down on the bed, I realized that the bed was like a rock—super immobile and hard. But in the end that was a very good thing. In two hours, I was supposed to address the Coast Guard troops.

The troops were very welcoming to me. I heard over and over, "Hip, hip, hooray!" as I walked all around them in the mess hall. Unfortunately for them, right behind me was a young, enlisted Coast Guard officer with a bucket—I threw up after every "Hip, hip, hooray!" Of course, everyone there knew that I was seasick and saw me

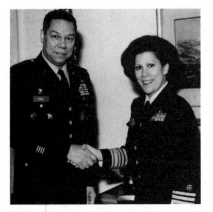

General Colin Powell, 65th US Secretary of State, shakes hands with Dr. Novello after awarding her the Legion of Merit.

vomit. I was so embarrassed but so seasick that all I wanted was to go onto the rock-hard bed—that wasn't moving—and rest.

The next morning, I was walking like John Wayne as I left the training ship. I kept walking that way for about a week. The things one does when duty calls. In the end, it was a great adventure.

General Colin Powell—who was serving when I served—and I were friends. He was from Jamaica, and I was from Puerto Rico. He would always say "Mira, Mira" to me, a very Puerto Rican greeting among friends. I always responded, "Don't try to mix—you are not a Puerto Rican, you are Jamaican," and we would both laugh.

One day he called me and said that he had to see me at the Pentagon where his office was, so I went. Suddenly, four or five men were marching with drums going into the hall and then into his office, just like in the movies, and I thought, *Oops, I'd better get back because I am in the middle of some important ceremony.* But to my surprise, the ceremony was meant for me. Colin Powell gave me the Legion of Merit. It was such a surprise and an honor since the services don't share medals among themselves and because the Legion of Merit is a very important and honorable award—and must be worn near the heart. I asked why I was receiving this award. I had forgotten that during the Kuwait War, he asked me to accelerate the anthrax vaccines through the FDA to get them to the military who were serving in the war. At that time, the director of the FDA was one of the Congressional Fellows who had been with me when we both worked for Senator Hatch. So I reached out to Dr. David Kessler and the process was finalized. The soldiers got their anthrax vaccines, and I got my medal.

I wondered out loud to my friend General Powell why we couldn't have a comparable medal for the Public Health Service Corps of Engineers who were able to take care of the oil fires in Kuwait. Colin Powell said, "We don't share medals. Go invent your own." So I did. There is now a ribbon and medal called the Crisis Response Service Award. Just because he dared me.

Dr. Albert B. Sabin, who helped develop the oral vaccine for polio, was also a very close friend. He had expressed his wish to be buried in Arlington National Cemetery even though he was not a military career officer. He was, however, a very important civilian. I am proud that I was able,—with the help of a few Senators—to get an extraordinary permission for him to be buried at Arlington. He is buried right next to Walter Reed on top of a little mountain.

While I was Surgeon General, it almost never happened that I could rest on an airplane. Basically, I would go in the back like everybody else, but when people saw me in my uniform, especially during the later years of my tenure, once they knew who I was, they often tried to move me up to first class.

My assistant, Lydia, and I were traveling to Puerto Rico, and we both got moved up to first class. Later, the flight attendant was frantically running up and down the aisle looking for a doctor. I raised my hand, but she looked at me and said, "I know that you are a political doctor, don't worry about it." But she found no other volunteers and came back to see me. Both Lydia and I took off our blue Public Health Service jackets and went to the back of the plane where a man who was in one of the middle seats appeared like he had fainted. I got him in the aisle and started to give him CPR. I requested and got from the flight attendant a blood pressure cuff, a stethoscope, and oxygen. Lydia handled the oxygen. I took his blood pressure. I thought he might have had a vasovagal reflex until I smelled him, and he reeked of alcohol. After a while, we concluded that he was truly drunk. At first, while I was straddling this man giving him CPR with my white uniform blouse and epaulettes on my shoulders, I guess I looked like any flight attendant doing her job. Someone came up to me and tapped me on the shoulder. This man asked me if I had taken the blood pressure correctly and I assured him that I had. The man said, "Is he okay?" I said, "Yes," and I got annoyed. And I said, "Sir, do you have a Valium?" He said, "A Valium, what do you need a Valium for?" And, I said, "It is not for him or for me, it is for you. Will you sit down?" He said, "I'm a physician." I said, "Sir, I am not a flight attendant. I am the Surgeon General of the United States, and where were you when the flight attendant was trying to find a doctor? Sit down." He sat down. When we landed, the man who had fainted was taken out to the ambulance. We got our jackets, were thanked by the Captain, and out we went. Just a normal day at the office.

On another occasion, I was going to Geneva, Switzerland. Although I was seated at the back of the plane, the flight attendant said, "I heard that you are the Surgeon General. We are going to move you up to first class." I was savoring the thought of six hours to Geneva: the food would be great, and I would get to rest and relax. That would not be the case. The flight attendant came to me and asked me to help her. There at the back of first class was a man in his seat with a lot of food in front of him. He told me he was having chest pain. I took his blood pressure. Not bad but not good, either. Just to make conversation and because the blood pressure cuff was so old, I asked him if he had ever felt like this before. He said, "Oh, yes, before they did my triple bypass." So perhaps one of his stents was clogged or he could be having a mild heart attack on the plane. I asked him if he had something that generally helped him in this situation. He said that he usually had nitroglycerin, but it hadn't happened in a long time, so he didn't have any medication with him. The pilot came for a consultation with me and asked me what I wanted to do. At this point, we were smack in the middle between Geneva and the United States. I told the pilot that I would keep monitoring the passenger and if there were a crisis, he would be alerted. I asked to have an ambulance waiting when we arrived in Geneva. I asked the passenger where he was going, and he told me that he had business in Africa and that he was giving a speech. Our plane was going to Geneva and then on to Africa. I monitored his blood pressure for the rest of the flight. We landed in Geneva, and I went to the front of the plane and began to fill out the paperwork for the ambulance. When I came back to tell him that everything was ready for him, he was gone. He had gone out of the back exit of the plane. I hope he survived.

* * *

I had the idea that something was wrong with my marriage, but I never truly asked or questioned it. The marriage had been limping, but it wasn't broken. But when I became Surgeon General, the marriage ruptured at the seams. I became consumed with my new job; I took very seriously both the nation's health and the average citizen. There were sacrifices to be made. And in the end, I made choices— based on the circumstances as I understood them. Maybe I wasn't paying enough attention to the ones in my house. Still today, I wonder how much I was to blame.

Or maybe Joe was just very good at keeping secrets. He had had a lover for many years, but I never knew about her until we were getting divorced. He was never late and never absent. I tried to compensate for my time out of the house and on the road. When I would take a California trip, for example, I would take the midnight flight and then come back on the redeye the next day. That way, I was there in the morning when he woke up. I also left food for him to eat. But I didn't feel that my efforts were appreciated. Of course, the food I left for him when I traveled was never eaten, but I just dismissed it. And we never had time to fight because I had a speech to do or a weekend visit someplace, and my life had become that of the Surgeon General.

Joe never really took my job as Surgeon General seriously. And to make things worse, he had to relinquish what he loved the most: his television career and his three-hour radio show, which he had had for the longest time—and Washington, D.C., adored it and him. Everyone knew the voice, and everybody knew the man. Both shows were terminated when I became Surgeon General because they were paid for by Pfizer Pharmaceutical, and it became a conflict of interest. Joe was devastated and lost his identity for a while. Here he was unhappy—he had a plane, he had a Mercedes, he had a house in a very expensive neighborhood in D.C., he had no children, and he was a catch. I think deep down in his heart he never truly recovered from these losses, and in his eyes, I was the culprit. Because now I was no longer three feet behind him, I was an equal. And maybe I wasn't paying enough attention to him.

One of those occasions was when Joe came home on a winter night and slipped on the ice on the sidewalk. He fractured his right arm. Unaware that I was home, he went alone to the emergency room at Georgetown Hospital. He came home late and in pain, but because at that time we were living in the same house, but on different floors, I didn't see him until morning. I am pretty sure that if the Surgeon General had taken him to the emergency room, the treatment would have happened more quickly, and I felt bad about that. Shortly thereafter, I left for Geneva for two weeks and left him at home alone with no use of his right arm. He couldn't cook or bathe or dress himself. To this day, I don't know how he survived, or why I left him alone when he needed my help. I felt guilty but realized that someone had helped him. He survived and I had a job to do. I have never forgotten that moment nor have I ever forgiven myself.

I often took one of my secretaries with me when I went to Puerto Rico. On one trip, I knew my accompanying secretary had a crush on the Admiral in charge of Roosevelt Roads Naval Base. So I told her,

"You know you are married, and you really shouldn't see him when you are traveling with me." She became enraged and asked why I should tell her what to do, especially since my husband wasn't behaving. I had deluded myself for so long, I didn't believe her when she told me of Joe's infidelities. She said she had been at the train station restaurant, and she saw Joe holding hands with a woman. And he saw her. This was the first time I had heard of his infidelities, and now here I was being scolded by my secretary. She was using Joe's infidelities against me and to excuse her own indiscretions. I was mortified, confused, lost, and sickened. It turned out the Admiral she had eyes on was dating other women also.

* * *

My husband, the psychiatrist, said the biggest primal scream he'd ever heard came from the bathroom at six o'clock in the morning on December 9, 1992. I had just heard on the radio that I was being replaced by the incoming President, Bill Clinton, with his current Director of the Arkansas Department of Health, Dr. Joycelyn Elders. When I recovered from the shock, Joe asked me, "What are you going to do about it?" And I said, "I don't know, you tell me." He replied, "What's on the agenda today?" And I said, "I am walking into one of those meetings today regarding tobacco—and I am already a lame duck." He said, "Well, what do you do when you see a patient who has cancer?" I responded with, "I just walk in there and deal with it." And he said, "That is exactly what you are going to do. It is not your problem, it is his."

Later that day, when I walked into the tobacco meeting, it was packed. I don't know why or what possessed me, but I walked into the room limping. So everybody came up to me and asked, "Dr. Novello, what is wrong?" I said, "I'm just a lame duck, but let's get the show on the road," and we did. It was very hard to do policy meetings that needed results when the results or their implementation were at risk of not occurring. I did this lame duck work from December 1992 through the end of June 1993.

Even though I heard the news about Joycelyn's appointment on December 9, it was not until December 23, as I was boarding a plane to Puerto Rico for Christmas vacation, that I got a call from Secretary of HHS Dr. Donna Shalala apologizing for getting hold of me so late since I was a career Public Health Officer. Secretary Shalala said she wanted me to keep the rank of three stars after I left the position. I thanked her, but I told her that there was only person with three stars and that was the Surgeon General.

Interestingly, when I returned from vacation in January of 1993, I was told that Dr. Elders was not coming until July because she was the President of the American Public Health Association through June 30. And I asked myself, why in the hell didn't they know this before they made me—the sitting Surgeon General—a lame duck? I guess no one had told them that the Surgeon General serves for a four-year term after appointment by the President and then confirmation by the US Senate. I was caught in the middle of people with power not knowing the basic rules regarding the Office of the Surgeon General.

Later, I learned that other Surgeons General who faced termination before the end of their four-year terms had political support that enabled them to stay longer. Dr. David Satcher had nine months left on his tenure when President Clinton left office and George W. Bush became President. The whole Black Caucus marched to the White House and asked that he be given the time to finish his four years. President Bush abided by the request and Dr. Satcher finished his tenure.

I had the same nine months left on my tenure as Dr. Satcher had had when I heard about Joycelyn's selection, but in my case, the Hispanic Caucus didn't march to the White House. Some members of that caucus instead called me to sign autographs and to take final pictures. It was very painful. But since I was a career officer of the Public Health Service and the President is the Chief of the Uniformed Services, I did what was expected of me.

During this time, I had the press on my back constantly. I told them not to confuse dignity with weakness—the President was my boss, and, as an officer, whatever he decided was okay with me. It was very hard to say that, but I would never say a bad word against the President. As a career officer, I always abided by the rules. Honestly, I was heartbroken, but I kept doing my job until the end.

Upon my impending departure as Surgeon General, the moving van was full of my furniture, my office was packed, and as a true public health career officer I was ready to move back to the NIH. That day I got my second call from Dr. Shalala. She was calling to tell me that I could not move that day because she had just gotten a call from the Senator from Massachusetts. His wife was a member of NIH in the Division of Mental Health. I was supposed to be moving into her old office, but the desk that was in her office was a family heirloom and she was afraid that if I moved in, it would be damaged. I was an angry lame duck again. I left everything packed and in the middle of my office. From that point until I was actually allowed to move into my office at the NIH—which wasn't for several months—I had two chairs in my office in front of the boxes and held all of my meetings there. Thereafter, I was assigned to UNICEF but kept my office at the NIH.

In 1994, I was at UNICEF Paris when Joe called me at two a.m. He said to turn on CNN. So I did, and there was President Clinton asking Joycelyn Elders to resign her post, only fifteen months into the job. Elders had endorsed a variety of positions that were deemed to be controversial. Her comments on masturbation led to President Clinton's request for her resignation.

At that moment, I thought being friends with the President was not a good thing. If he had really cared for her as Surgeon General, the way he had talked about her as Health Commissioner in Arkansas, he would have let her stay in her job twenty-one more days. This would have been a kind gesture for history. Then she would have

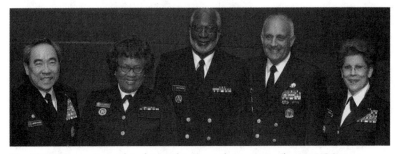

Five US Surgeons General. Left to right: *Kenneth Moritsugu (acting US Surgeon General), Dr. Joycelyn Elders, Dr. David Satcher, Dr. Richard Carmona, and Dr. Antonia Novello.*

appeared to have served from 1993 to 1995 and she would never have had to explain the shortness of her tenure.

After she was fired, Joycelyn and I became very close. We both have scars from the position that we served. We were both naive and trusting when we entered the job as Surgeon General, both of us just trying to save the world. And we both got quite an education while we were in the position.

CHAPTER 7

UNICEF and Beyond

Since I was leaving the office of Surgeon General but was still an officer of the Public Health Service, I had to be placed in a position commensurate with my rank. I was supposed to be sent to the World Health Organization (WHO) rather than UNICEF at the end of my term as Surgeon General, but the US had plans to remove the WHO Director at the time and decided to not have me go through another political mishap. I arrived at UNICEF in mid-1993.

UNICEF was quite an experience, but after being Surgeon General, it was hard to be Special Assistant to the Director in areas that I felt were too simple for my expertise. My arrogance was unlimited. The Director was Mr. Grant who had been there for years and was adored. He was the ultimate diplomat—knowledgeable and kind. Everyone he met was treated with the same respect as the President.

When Mr. Grant told me that he wanted me to help iodize the salt of the world, I must have looked at him like: Are you kidding me? I had been the Surgeon General. Have you ever heard of Morton's Salt? I was not amused. So I said, "If you will give me an explanation of why iodization of salt is important to you, then maybe I will be able to help you."

Mr. Grant said that the lack of iodine is the biggest cause of mental disability in the world. And at moments when there are dictators and presidents abusive toward and controlling of their people, they will use a lack of iodine as a weapon to control the populace by removing it from the food supply. All of a sudden, I decided that this was more important than anything I had ever heard. I was adamant that everyone in the world would have iodized salt for their citizens. So I went ahead and helped iodize everything I could get my hands on. The first country was China, whose interest in iodizing their salt was spurred by the one-child policy and by the fact that Mr. Grant had been born there as his parents were missionaries.

An invitation came to him to speak at the Forbidden City in Beijing about giving iodine to the People's Republic of China. When he couldn't go, he called me and asked if I had my passport with me. When I said, "Yes," he said, "Good, because you will be getting on a plane tonight for China." I thought, *What, you've got to be kidding!* He said, "You're going to China. You're going to give my speech. Don't worry, it has been written on my behalf. All you have to do is go to the Hall of the Forbidden City and give it."

So I went to China. They called my name to come to the microphone, and I swear to God, I could not see the last person in the last row because there were just rows and rows of people, extending forever—as far as the eye could see. This speech, of course, was to ensure that we would iodize the salt of China—for all people, including the minorities; I was giving Mr. Grant's mandate. The people of China held him in such high regard because he had been born there. At the end, all the applause was not for me but for Mr. Grant. China iodized its salt faster than any other country, which was facilitated by the type of government they have.

What happened after my speech was a surprise. When I was done, we proceeded to the place where Mao Tse Tung used to hold meetings. The two chairs used by Mao were there as was his spittoon, which was to my right. I was in one of the chairs and the Financial Minister was on my left in the other. And I kept noticing that despite how strong communism was at that time in China, the Financial Minister was wearing a Hermes designer tie and belt and Ferragamo shoes—not quite the accessories that Mao Tse Tung himself would have worn and certainly not made in China!

When I was out in Beijing in a car, I remember being surrounded by so many bicycles. Thousands of bicycles. Everyone was eating in front of little shops, with smoke rising from the cooking units. In the parks, people—mostly the elderly—were doing tai chi. I then was taken to the Great Wall of China.

My female interpreter was looking at my clothes during my entire visit. I decided something at the end of the day: this woman had been so good to me that I would give her the clothes I was wearing; I had an extra skirt and blouse in my purse. I gave her my blouse, my skirt, and my belt. I thought she was going to die of happiness. I certainly couldn't give her American dollars because that would have been unacceptable, so she got my clothes.

I bought some beautiful vases—blue ceramics in the old part of Beijing—and put them in my carry-on. Unfortunately, we flew to Hong Kong on Air India and there was a typhoon. The other items I had bought in China were in my suitcase. Many of them had red ink and, when my suitcase got soaking wet, the ink bled and ruined all my clothes. But the vases were safe. To this day they are in my house as a memory of my visit to China as a guest of the Chinese government.

The next country where we iodized the salt was India. Because cows are sacred in India, we had to iodize the salt fed to cows before we could iodize the salt fed to humans. The iodized salt campaign worked as well in India as it had in China. Then one country after another did their job, and we finalized our tasks regarding the children's agenda pertaining to iodization in less than five years.

Mr. Grant was very forceful in advocating for the poor—especially treatments for diarrhea, dehydration, and hunger, and he wanted to make the treatment for them affordable. He addressed many groups, and I accompanied him to many of these talks.

For example, if he wanted to save the children from diarrhea and dehydration, he would pull out of his jacket a small package that when dissolved in water would serve as nutrients—almost like intravenous fluids—and the cost was no more than 5 cents.

If he wanted to address responsible sexual encounters and protection against HIV/AIDS, he would pull out a condom and give a preventive talk.

Everything was going well—until he started talking about breastfeeding. He wanted every mother to be taught how to breastfeed. For the life of me, I always feared that he would make me take my breast out and show how. Obviously, it was at this time that I decided to carefully screen where I was going with him and what the topic was going to be.

Also during my time with UNICEF, I met His Holiness John Paul—the Polish Pope. I went to see him with the former governor of Florida. Little groups have visits with the Pope to minimize the number of interviews he must do. To meet with him, women must have a hair covering. The cardinals had long gowns and all kinds of chains hanging on their chests. They guided us, accompanying us from room to room until there we were—with the Pope. He stood, and we were to greet him, genuflect, and kiss his hand. He knew Spanish. So I said, Father, I see you have lost a little bit of weight." And he said, "Espanola, ah? Only a Spanish woman can come up to me to tell me that I have lost weight." He then gave us rosaries, and we were guided out. I met him maybe four times during my UNICEF years because the Vatican supported many of the UNICEF initiatives, and in addition, we always gave speeches during the Vatican's yearly conference. What humanity the Pope displayed each time I met him. I was devastated when he died—but I was glad he was canonized by the church.

After Mr. Grant died in early 1995, a new Director was brought in to run UNICEF who did not have Mr. Grant's tact and/or diplomacy. I was glad the time had come for me to go back to the NIH.

* * *

All the frustrations and perhaps the newly acknowledged infidelities were too much for us both to bear—so my marriage came to an end. Joe had been sleeping upstairs since 1990. He had asked me for a divorce the first time in 1990 on one of our walks through the neighborhood. But my niece was living with us then. It wasn't a good time to move forward with a divorce, so the matter was dropped, and the marriage limped along. In 1992, when I came back from one of my trips to California, Joe had left me a succinct note that said, "I'm leaving, I can't take this anymore." And he left the house. I filed for divorce and submitted the paperwork. I felt it was time I freed myself from so many uncertainties and so many lies.

I finally admitted Joe's infidelities around the time we were getting divorced. I asked his secretary if she knew anything about his infidelities. She said that every Monday a different woman's voice would call on the telephone for him. I asked her to please tell me when she heard from these women, so that I would not be embarrassed when I was in a public place and one of those women could be laughing at me.

I forgot to make dinner reservations for Joe's forty-ninth birthday and, in anger, he moved to the fourth-floor bedroom. During our twenty-four years of marriage, I had always put together some sort of celebration. For example, for his fortieth birthday, there were forty people at a black-tie dinner at the Hay Adams Hotel, complete with the violin music that he loved. But in 1991, when he turned fifty, not forty-nine, and expected a huge party with favors and dancing with all his friends in a great hall, he was gravely disappointed. Instead, I invited his five favorite couples. We had chateaubriand, champagne, and cake, and I gave him a Cartier gold watch (which took me three years to pay off) to celebrate the day. He didn't want the watch. He didn't enjoy the party, and he did not appreciate the small scale for his fiftieth.

We got divorced in 1994. But the judge decided, and Joe requested, that since our house had four levels and an elevator and because Joe was supposed to continue paying the mortgage, we would each have one floor to ourselves, and we would share the rest of the house. We did that from 1994 through 1998, when the house finally sold. The divorce became final at that point.

During the four years that we lived in the same house awaiting its sale, Joe was always asking me what my plans were regarding marriage. I told him none. I had lost all my trust in him. I lived on the second floor; he lived on the fourth floor. He tried to cook once, but he made such a mess. I then decided to do the cooking because I didn't want to deal with the chaos. So for about four years, I was the one who was maintaining what might have looked like a regular household routine.

During the division of our furniture, I gave him everything he wanted. The dining room set. All the china. The bedroom furniture. The kitchen utensils. I could not understand why he wanted all the things that usually went to the wife. I only kept the living room furniture and the guest bedroom furniture. There was a house that we had at one point planned to move into from our Georgetown house; instead, Joe moved there with the woman whom he had been having an affair with for twenty years. In the end, he did not marry her, he married the neighbor instead.

As we were leaving the Georgetown house, I came across many things that Joe would have liked. I asked his secretary if we could take them to his house—to which she responded, "No," very harshly. "Don't you know that this man doesn't love you?" What an eye opener for me. The secretary had more power than his wife and knew more than I did about what he needed.

It was eerie during the reading of the divorce decree. My lawyer said she had never met a man who loved his wife more and was still divorcing her. That day, I needed to pick up the Minister of Health of Nicaragua at noon as I was working for UNICEF at the time and that was part of my duty. In my rush to leave, I heard that Joe had $450,000 in assets between bonds, cash, coins, and silver. At the same time, I heard that I had antiques valued at $450,000 as well—therefore he was to keep the money and I was to keep the antiques. I could not believe it. Antiques that I paid maybe $87,000 for had been valued at $450,000 and appraised without my permission or knowledge? And worse, that sum would be deducted from the final funds I was to get from the sale of the house.

Unbeknownst to me, Joe had gone to the shop where I had purchased the antiques and requested an appraisal of them. The owner loved Joe and the antiques, which had belonged to her, and exaggerated the price thinking that it was only an appraisal—nothing else. Because the $450,000 value of the antiques was then deducted from the sale of the house, as were all the home improvements and modifications we had made over the years, I had only $400,000 left from the sale of $1,550,000. I used this as the down payment for my Watergate condominium.

It was not a pleasant divorce, and Joe spent very little money on his attorney because, as luck would have it, when he left the house before the judge allowed him to come back (since he didn't want to pay the extra rent when he had a mortgage to pay), his roommate was the Chairman of the law firm that handled his end of the divorce. I had to pay $21,000 of the money I had gotten in the settlement to my lawyer and Joe's divorce was free. So I ended up moving into the Watergate and then started my job in New York State as the Health Commissioner in 1999.

I didn't tell anyone I was divorced from Joe because I didn't think it was their business. I didn't even tell my mother for a whole year because she would have said that I failed. Mami thought Joe was the perfect individual, and then all of a sudden, I had failed at marriage? When I got to Puerto Rico to tell her, unbeknownst to me, she had moved to a different house—so I couldn't even find her at first! When I finally told her, it was devastating to her and devastating for me to remember it. Mami loved Joe very much, and I believe she must have been in communication with him to ask him what went wrong.

Mami came to visit me after the divorce was final when I was living at Watergate. Since she and Joe had continued their communication, I invited Joe to meet us at a restaurant for lunch. At the time, I was writing my thesis for my doctorate in public health. After the lunch he came to my place at Watergate and saw the introduction that I was drafting that included the acknowledgments. I had given it to him to read because he was a wonderful writer and editor. He saw that his name was not mentioned. I know that that was very hurtful for him. But he didn't remember that he had never dedicated one of his books to me either, that I was always included in a group of people in the acknowledgments.

One of Joe's very close friends called me while I was at my Watergate apartment. This friend was so sympathetic to Joe, commiserating that I had been frigid, that Joe and I had never had any intimacy, that Joe could not be blamed for looking for somebody that he loved and wanted to marry. All without hearing my side of the story. How could I share with a stranger who accused me of frigidity that I had my personal reasons? How could I sleep with a man whose penis could have been anywhere the night before? All our friends took Joe's side. Because I never talked about Joe's and my private life, they just assumed that I was at fault. I have never regained any of those friendships. Joe was also very good at portraying himself as the victim. Even Mom and Dad Novello must have believed him, since I was not invited to his niece's wedding, and I was not invited to their sixtieth wedding anniversary celebration either. His girlfriend was—I saw her in the pictures.

A single woman at a dinner is competition, but a single man is an asset.

I haven't really allowed myself to date since the divorce. I did see one person for about a year and a half; he was a companion. This companionship made me realize almost fifteen years postdivorce how much I needed affection and a human touch. After a while, though, I realized that the relationship was not working. Again, I found myself giving too much and getting very little in return. So it ended. It was another lesson learned—thank God that the biggest mistakes are often for the shortest duration.

But that was the only time that I saw someone other than Joe. I didn't want to make my life miserable, and I was certainly not going to be a nurse or a purse; no man should expect me to come into his life to take care of all his ailments. Doctor for the world, yes. But not an in-house nurse for a husband. What a fool I was. Life has a way of showing you how you can be wrong.

* * *

When I was working on my doctorate in public health at Johns Hopkins University, my thesis was "The Modern Era, Surgeons General." For my thesis, I had to do a compilation of all the surviving Surgeons General, and then I presented a proposal to the Dean. The Dean wanted me to get all the Surgeons General together to do a lecture that would be called "The Future of Health Care in This Nation." He said it would be a great thing for the university, that he would cancel any class that was scheduled during that time, and that all the students would be invited to listen, either in the amphitheater or piped into other rooms. Would that be okay?

Well, once I commit to anything in my life, I practically kill myself to see that it happens. I called every single surviving Surgeon General, but my big worry was how to entice Dr. Koop to come. When I called him, I said, "Dr. Koop, I am doing a symposium where all of the surviving Surgeons General are going to talk about the health of the nation for the future, and I want to invite you." And he said, "Let me look at my calendar. Well, Toni, the only day I have available in the coming year [1998] is the second of April." And I said, "Dr. Koop, you aren't going to believe this, but that is exactly the day that I had scheduled for the symposium." Now he was trapped and could not say no. And I used the date and the fact Dr. Koop was attending to invite all of the others.

Nevertheless, after Dr. Koop, I did have some difficulty with the two oldest Surgeons General. One was deaf, so everyone in the university knew I was inviting him as I was screaming into the phone. The second one told me he couldn't come because he had church choir practice that day. In the end, each of their wives came to the phone, and I was able to converse with them and get commitments for both of their husbands to attend.

As it turned out, all the surviving Surgeons General attended. The more recent ones wore their uniforms; the older ones did not. I met for the first time the Surgeon Generals of Presidents Eisenhower, Nixon, Johnson, and Carter. The place was packed with students from the School of Public Health and from the medical school. So many questions. So much interest. I had also invited former US Attorney General Janet Reno to the symposium, and she gave the closing remarks.

The Dean was so appreciative that he gave the Dean's Medal of Hopkins to each of us. He sponsored a lovely lunch before the symposium for all of us as well, where we caught up on each other's news. And the photos that were taken of the US Surgeons General were used by Hopkins as their Christmas card that year for their alumni. It also became the start of periodic gatherings of the Surgeons General to talk about public policy and health, wherever and whenever the need arose.

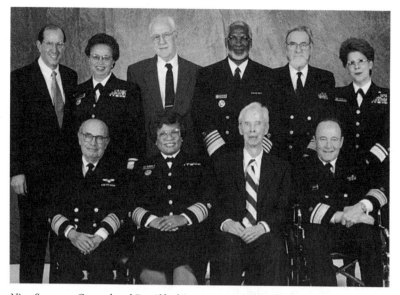

Nine Surgeons General and Dr. Alfred Sommer at Johns Hopkins University, April 2, 1998, at a celebration for the 200th anniversary of the US Public Health Service and the 50th anniversary of the Declaration of Human Rights. Standing from left to right: Dr. Alfred Sommer, Dean of the Johns Hopkins Bloomberg School of Public Health; Audrey F. Manley, MD, MPH; William Steward, MD; David Satcher, MD, PhD; C. Everett Koop, MD, ScD; and Antonia Novello, MD, MPH, DrPH. Seated from left to right: Julius B. Richmond, MD, MS; M. Joycelyn Elders, MD, MS; Leroy E. Burney, MD, MPH; and S. Paul Ehrlich, Jr. MD, MPH. Photo courtesy of Johns Hopkins Bloomberg School of Public Health.

CHAPTER 8

So Much More Than Vaccines

After being the Surgeon General, I had never considered being the Commissioner of Health of a state. I thought all those jobs entailed were vaccinations, inspections, and health messages. Plus, after serving as US Surgeon General, I thought that sort of job was not for me.

But I was wrong. Little did I know that my perception of the job would change drastically.

In 1998, I was invited to Seneca Falls, New York, to give the keynote speech at an event honoring the 150th anniversary of the beginning of the fight for women's rights. I had been inducted into the National Women's Hall of Fame based in Seneca Falls in 1994 and returned periodically when invited. I had just moved from my house in Georgetown. I had packed two suitcases—one, which was meant for the laundry, was to go to the house where I would be staying after the divorce and before Watergate, the other was to go to Seneca Falls.

To my surprise and dismay, after I arrived in Seneca Falls, when I went to iron my clothes for my speech, I discovered that I had picked up the wrong suitcase! Most of the clothes were for informal gatherings and were going to the laundry upon my return. I picked out the least smelly and the only pantsuit there in which I could look even semi-presentable. I was truly upset. But my assistant's clothes, which were offered, were not my size and neither were the clothes offered by the Chairwoman of the meeting. Maybe no one noticed my attire, but I certainly knew it and felt that I was not at my best. I think the reception to the speech helped erase the agony that I felt about not being in top form.

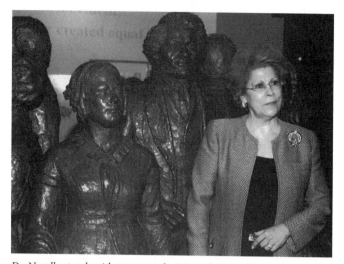

Dr. Novello stands with statues at the Women's Rights National Historical Park in Seneca Falls, New York.

It turned out that the Chairwoman of the meeting was also the Chairperson of the New York State Public Health Council. She said she needed my CV, as the job of Commissioner of the Department of Health of the State of New York was vacant, and she wanted to recommend me to the Governor. Which she did. Due to her recommendation, I had lunch in New York City with a woman who had been a special advisor to the Governor. As luck would have it, at the same time, I was being asked to run for the position of Mayor of San Juan, Puerto Rico.

Pedro Rosselló served as Governor of Puerto Rico from 1993 to 2001. A fellow physician, we always liked each other. I spent many nights in La Fortaleza—the Governor's Residence—in the Kennedy Room. One night in 1998 when I was in Washington, D.C., I went to dinner with his press secretary who informed me that the Governor wanted to see me. When I asked why, the press secretary said he didn't know but felt that it was important. The Governor and I had participated in many forums together, and when I was no longer the Surgeon General, he asked me to be his Secretary of Health. I thanked him but did not accept. To me, it was too much of a step down to go from being Surgeon General of the United States to being Puerto Rico Health Secretary, so I declined. Arrogance to the fullest!

Now I was intrigued by what he had in mind for me. I went to Puerto Rico with Joe and met with the Governor. To my surprise, he offered me the post of Mayor of San Juan. This was a post that was a rung on the ladder to the governorship of Puerto Rico, and I was honored that he had asked me. I said I would accept if I knew I could help him in his next term. Everything went well until, as we were leaving his office, the Governor said, "Tonita, do not limit your thinking only to the office of Mayor." "What the hell did he mean?" Joe asked. I had almost agreed to go with the job of Mayor, and now he was talking about paying attention to something else as well. We were confused. Time was of the essence.

The campaign team came forward. We met, we had a fight song, and there was a cadre of people who were going to help me run. The campaign had put together collateral that had my face everywhere—in pictures, banners, and so forth—hanging from walls. Budgets were in place—everything.

We had a meeting of the campaign team, and I asked a few questions: Before the elections, who will pay my salary? Where would I live? Who would help write my speeches? Who would oversee my daily campaign routine? To whom do I report? What are the important issues that need to be addressed?

The answer to all these questions was, "Doctora, it will be solved." "Doctora, it will come into view." This gave me no confidence in the approach, and as I told them: "If I were a male candidate for Mayor, would you give him the same answers that you have given me?" They all suggested that I had to do it for Puerto Rico. I told them to give me twenty-four hours to make my decision, and I went back home to D.C. The campaign group was not happy, and they kept telling me that I had to do this for my country.

Almost immediately after my departure, the Puerto Rican newspapers announced that the Governor was not going to run for another four-year term. Now I understood what he was saying to me the day we met at his office. I flew back to Puerto Rico, met with the team, and told them I was sorry but that I was not going to run for Mayor. All hell broke loose. They were in shock. I left the island with deep compassion for all those Representatives and Senators who had wanted me to be Mayor. But I felt they had not been true to me or to my prospective future. Similarly, I was feeling somewhat bad that they did not want me to have any contact with the previous Governor, who was a woman and a friend of mine. I felt uneasy already about people trying to curtail my liberty.

When I got home that night from Puerto Rico, I contacted the woman who had been such a significant supporter of mine and rather pushy about me running for Mayor. I wanted to explain to her my personal and more deeply felt reasons for not accepting the office. It was late at night when I called her at home. Her son answered and said she couldn't come to the phone. She was having a conversation with the former President of the Puerto Rico Senate—trying to convince him to run for Mayor! Less than twenty-four hours after she had begged me to "do it for your country."

After I hung up the phone, I opened an express delivery letter that had apparently arrived that day. It was a letter from the State of New York asking me to interview for the job of Health Commissioner. An opportunity truly beckoned. Although I had sent a certified letter to the assistant to the Governor thanking him for the opportunity, I had said thanks but no thanks when I was considering running for the position of Mayor of San Juan. Surprisingly, the assistant to the Governor had read the letter but never delivered it to the Governor. When one door closes, there is always another that opens in its place.

I traveled to Albany to be interviewed for the job by Governor George Pataki's Chief of Staff. Legislative hearings were necessary

> **"When one door closes, there is always another that opens in its place."**

for my confirmation. Time was of the essence because the New York legislature would stop meeting in two days, and then it would be six months before I could be confirmed. So I interviewed for the job. I went on a cold, gray, and unwelcoming day. I had never been to Albany before and as a native Puerto Rican, contrary to many people's beliefs, I had been in the State of New York only a few times in my life and I was only eight years old.

The Governor's Chief of Staff interviewed me and inquired about why I wanted this job. But in reality, I didn't want it! So I said we all had a little bit of Pollyanna inside and believed that some good might come out of situations like this one. And I reminded him that they had contacted me, not the other way around.

Then I interviewed with Governor Pataki. His Public Affairs Director came in. She thought the Governor did not look well and said so to him in language like, "You look like shit!" At first, I thought she was referring to me, but she was talking about him. Apparently, she was known for this kind of talk, but in time, I realized that she was also excellent at her job. Meanwhile, I indicated that I was a doctor and that I would be willing to take a look at him if he was interested. There was a stethoscope framing an award hanging on the wall, I removed it, and I did an examination and determined that he had pneumonia. He said, "I'm okay. I have bronchitis." And, I said, "Sir, do you have a doctor I can call?" He said, "I have one, and I am supposed to go see him, but I haven't had the time." I said, "Give me the number." And I called the doctor. I told him that the Governor either had severe bronchitis or pneumonia, but that he was not well. Governor Pataki got dressed and went to see his doctor. His doctor called me and thanked me—Governor Pataki had pneumonia. For as long as I was Commissioner (June 1999 through January 2007), every time Governor Pataki got sick, I would be called.

We had to hurry. When I asked what I should do since it looked like the job might be mine, I was told that I should go and talk to the President of the Senate, Senator Joseph Bruno, as he was the one who had to schedule my hearing.

I found the office of Senator Bruno and learned he was not there—he was giving a press conference. I had learned a few tricks of the trade over the years, so I waited at the closed door where the press conference was being held. When the door opened, I knew that the Senator would be running out with reporters in tow. The door opened and the first one out I felt was Senator Bruno. I identified myself as Dr. Novello and told him that my fate was in his hands. If he allowed hearings to be held, I might be appointed the next New York State Health Commissioner.

Senator Bruno was very intrigued by the name Novello, finding a commonality in surnames with Italian origins and believing that Italians could do good work. He scheduled the hearings, I testified, and then I watched the proceedings from the balcony as Senator Bruno proposed me for Health Commissioner. I was confirmed by all members except one woman and one man. The woman hurriedly came up to me after the hearing to inform me that voting against me was not personal—but that it was due to the issue of politics and abortion. I was just beginning to understand the politics involved in being a Commissioner in the state of New York. I was the second US Surgeon General to serve as Commissioner of Health of the State of New York as well—the first was Dr. Thomas Parran who served in the 1930s. But I was different from Dr. Parran—I was from the island of Puerto Rico, not from the Bronx, and the first Latino in the job.

The first thing I did in my job was visit each subdivision of the department. I met every person in the state of New York who worked for me. I shook every one of those hands. I was from Puerto Rico, and lots of people from Puerto Rico lived in the state. I wanted them all to realize that I was not only Commissioner but also a person who really knew public health and that I cared about them.

The building that housed the department was ugly and discombobulated. When I first entered, there were two people without any uniforms sitting at a puny little table with a bunch of cables coming out from under their feet. They were meant to be in charge of security. This is what people saw when they first entered the building. I walked a lot of corridors to get to my office and found it had a gated door. Apparently, the former Commissioner was not well-liked by AIDS activists, there had been an incident, and there was a need to protect her from the public.

Later, as I started feeling more accustomed to the job, I found the office of the Director who was in charge of funding building renovations. I asked him to help me get my office and my department in better shape than it was at the time I arrived. He asked me how much I needed, and I told him I didn't know—that I needed an engineer to evaluate it. It took months to redo the department, but it got done. The secretaries were placed in areas outside their bosses' offices. The conference room was redone with glass walls so that people could see that work was being done. And the reception area was modified so it wasn't just a table with wires coming out of it. In addition, there were no longer double doors separating the Commissioner from the public.

The New York State Department of Health is one-third of the entire New York state's budget. The department oversaw wide-ranging functions, from nursing homes to organ transplants to undertakers to tobacco. During my tenure, there were close to thirteen major episodes to deal with, including the collapsing towers of September 11, 2001.

During my first month as Commissioner, New York experienced the largest *E. coli* outbreak in the United States—second only to the 1992–1993 Jack-in-the-Box outbreak in California, Idaho, Washington, and Nevada. *E. coli* is a bacterium of the stools that when ingested—which usually happens with undercooked meat or contaminated water—can cause kidneys to shut down. I am a physician first, a pediatrician, and a nephrologist, so I said to the Governor, "I'm going to take this on my own."

New York is famous for petting zoos at fairs during the summer. The twenty-one children infected with *E. coli* had all been to a petting zoo at the county fair. So I went to the fair. I walked the whole county fair, and I was shown the water pump that was probably responsible for infecting the water people were drinking. The farmers at the fair told me that one infected cow can infect the water supply. Anyone drinking out of the water fountain fed by the pump could have gotten infected.

After a press conference to answer reporters' questions about the outbreak, I asked to meet with the parents. I said, "Get me the amphitheater at the hospital [Albany Medical]. I have walked the fair, the department staff has briefed me, and I will meet all the parents of these children there." The parents came to the amphitheater. I explained what I knew about the reason their children had gotten infected, and I made them a promise. I told them: "Every day at five o'clock, I will come here—and you will come here—and I will tell you exactly what I know about the infection, and I will tell you exactly what is going to happen to your children. At six o'clock, you will hear the same thing on the news, but I will always tell you first."

Because of this, such trust was built between the parents and me. One pregnant mother even named her son Anthony in my honor. Unfortunately, all twenty-one of the children developed renal failure, and they all needed dialysis. One of them was very, very sick—he probably developed chronic renal failure. No parent sued the Health Department, and twenty children survived. One little girl died, and a scholarship was established at one of the New York City schools of medicine in her name. At age three, she had already voiced the desire to be a doctor. Her mother would not bury her daughter until she had her CTR ring (a Mormon ring with the motto Choose the Right inscribed on it). Fortunately, I had been given a CTR ring when I worked for Senator Hatch, who was Mormon. I gave my ring to the little girl's mother, and they were able to bury their daughter in peace.

I kept a very close eye on all the petting zoos in New York for the rest of my tenure.

After *E. coli*, we had West Nile Virus. Then we had H1N1 and then SARS, then a shortage of influenza vaccines. Something was always happening.

Also during my first month on the job, I asked to attend and speak at a national meeting in Albany about HIV. HIV at the time was a political hot potato. The Governor's Public Affairs Director and first assistant both said, "No, you are not going to speak." And I replied, "Oh, yes, I'm going." After a little more back and forth, they said, "Well you're going to have a policeman behind you and you're going to go through the kitchen." I said that I wasn't going to have a police escort and that I wasn't going through the kitchen. "I haven't done anything wrong. I just got here."

I went. I walked in through the front of the conference. The HIV leaders gave me five minutes; I spoke from my heart and got a standing ovation. There was one thing I had learned. The HIV community is very close. They have a great network. If they like you, they will like you for life. If they don't like you, you are doomed. They knew I had done the HIV #2 report when I was Surgeon General. They also knew I had hung the AIDS quilt in my office. I had no problem with the HIV community or the gay community. I became an advocate for them and worked on their behalf during my entire time as the Commissioner. And I still do.

The politics of being the New York State Health Commissioner were brought home to me soon after the start of my tenure with the closing of an abortion clinic. The community was in an uproar, and every woman in the community was against the closure and blamed me personally, especially because I was a Catholic girl from Puerto Rico. Believing as I do so strongly in data and facts and transparency, I invited the women leaders to come see me—and they did.

I explained the facts of our investigation. These showed that many women came daily to the clinic for abortions. And even though at the time New York City had a very high HIV/AIDS infection rate, at this clinic, the white piece of paper covering the stretcher where an abortion was performed was not being fully removed or cleaned before the next abortion was performed. That created a significant risk of HIV/AIDS infection for the client. Similarly, there was only one very outdated (probably 1950s-era) blood pressure cuff that had to suffice for at least twenty patients, and only one manometer, to measure the blood pressure of the twenty or so patients. Each patient should have had her own blood pressure monitor to detect if she had gone into shock after the procedure. In addition, the abortion suction instrument being used was outdated, thereby causing undue pain. For all these reasons, I closed the clinic and gave it the opportunity to remedy the faults before it would be allowed to reopen.

The women in the community listened and understood the reasons and became very comfortable with the closure. In the end, it wasn't the Health Department that prolonged the closure of the clinic but the Mayor of New York City. Politics rearing its head again. The facility did finally reopen, ready to perform abortions as a decent, clean, and operational clinic.

During my tenure, quite a few doctors lost their licenses to practice because of irresponsible behavior or incompetence. A few of these cases were unique and memorable.

A neurosurgeon forgot to take the patient's MRIs into the operating room. Consequently, he operated on the wrong side of the patient's brain. In addition, he dropped one of the scalpels, which inadvertently made an incision in the spinal cord and some of the spinal fluid came out. When I found out that this was the second time he had done this, I felt he was not demonstrating care or respect for his patients, so his case was sent to the Physician's Conduct subdivision for review. The neurosurgeon lost his medical license and, in addition, was required to take extra education. I hoped he might learn some humility in the process as well.

Another case I won't forget centered around an autistic child. He always smelled of urine after his visits to his therapist. The department discovered the therapist was actually urinating on this child. The therapist's license was revoked.

Then there was the case where the urologist removed the wrong kidney from an elderly cancer patient—even with the explanation of which kidney to remove right in the front of the chart. The patient developed renal failure and died. Even though the pathology specimen showed that the good kidney, and not the bad one, had been removed, the doctor took no action. The committee that judged medical negligence decided that since he was a young urologist, he should be given a second chance, to which I said publicly, "Over my dead body. Who will return this father to his family?" I didn't believe he should be granted a second chance. Eventually, he made another mistake, and his medical license was finally revoked.

There was the pediatrician who performed physicals on female adolescents over the age of twelve with no one else in the room. After several complaints came in from his patients who were now adult women who, after they were married, realized his behavior was really sexual abuse, I was able to pull his license. He did not contest.

The death of a liver donor occurred over a Fourth of July weekend after a transplantation at a prestigious hospital in New York City. The liver donor was a reporter with a newspaper in Albany, and the recipient was his brother, who was a doctor in New York. The operation went very well. Over the holiday weekend, there was one intern and one fellow for all the patients who had undergone transplantations but no apparent visit by the chief transplant surgeon. The donor, who was now without part of his liver and his gallbladder, was nevertheless inappropriately fed lobster with butter the night after the operation. A person cannot digest that type of food without a gallbladder and worse less than one day after major liver surgery. He started vomiting dark brown material. It meant something was very wrong. He also got a bacterial infection. The medical fellow on duty proceeded to do a physical examination on the next transplant recipient for the morning after but not on the donor who was vomiting. The donor died. His brother lived.

I closed the transplantation unit. The fellow was taken off the case and sent for more training. The chief transplant surgeon was dismissed by the hospital and the intern abandoned the internship. As a result of this case, a committee was formed to oversee organ transplants and donors. Several years after this, all the Surgeons General were invited to speak at the International Transplant Society of the US about the lack of organs in the minority community. To my surprise, the President of the organization was the chief transplantation surgeon who had been dismissed because of that liver transplant case. Although we had a few awkward moments before the conference, during our conversations he agreed that I had done the right thing. Today he is an excellent surgeon doing a great job, and I am at peace with my decision.

Yes, under my leadership doctors' licenses were taken away. And yes, under my leadership hospitals were closed. My philosophy was to tell the truth. Every time I closed a hospital or took a doctor's license away, I went public and explained why. It is important to share the knowledge and explain exactly what had happened and why. That way, others could put themselves in my position and understand why I had made the decisions I did.

After almost a year on the job, I was asked to talk to the doctors of New York State to report on why I had taken some of their peers' licenses. Before I spoke to the group, the doctors' lobbyist begged me to keep it simple and light—not to mention the license removals.

How little he knew me. I started by addressing the reason for each removal, and I explained that since New York City was referred to as the "Big Apple," one rotten apple will damage all of us.

The audience understood. They applauded and from then on, I was invited to their meetings. Transparency in political jobs is of the utmost importance. It helps establish trust, which is the ultimate goal for survival.

* * *

In 1998, Joe developed a symptomatology that ended up being diagnosed as cancer of the prostate. He had been treating it as if it were an infection, but when I told him it might be cancer, he went to see a urologist friend of his. I was now Commissioner of Health in New York, and I got a call from Joe's secretary telling me that he wanted an appointment at Johns Hopkins because the best surgeon for prostate cancer, Dr. Patrick Walsh, was there. I called Dr. Walsh, who said he could not perform the surgery on Joe. As luck would have it, I was scheduled to be the keynote speaker for commencement at the medical school at Johns Hopkins. So I called the Dean and said if he wanted a speaker for commencement, then Dr. Walsh needed to do that surgery on Joe. Dr. Walsh called me. He wanted to know what I wanted and proceeded to tell me that Joe was seeing his partner and that he didn't feel it was appropriate to take patients from his partners. In the end, Dr. Walsh did perform the surgery on Joe, and it was successful.

The process involved for the prostate surgery was new to both me and Joe. Patients had the surgery in the hospital but stayed at a hotel nearby prior to the surgery. Then, after being released from intensive care postsurgery, they returned to the hotel. I had reserved the hotel as Joe had requested, and I asked him if he wanted me to stay the night before with him. He responded, "Toni, I have to tell you something. I'm seeing someone. She will be there, and she has the right." I went numb.

After the shock of the moment, I recall two things—I was in my office in New York, and there were many people waiting to see me outside my office, but fortunately, the door was closed. I was blank in disbelief. I knew there were infidelities but putting me aside like a useless instrument in his life (after I had arranged for everything) was too much to bear. I told him, "Joe, I can't believe you." Then I hung up the phone, removed my wedding rings, and threw them in the garbage. That was the true end of my innocence and our marriage. I called his parents, told them what Joe had done, and assured them that, despite everything, he would do well and that I would continue to help. The day of his surgery, all his cousins, friends, and family were there, but I was not. His girlfriend was at his bedside.

When the surgery was completed, Dr. Walsh called me first and told me about the successful operation—as he didn't know that Joe and I were divorced. The surgery was around Memorial Day. When the Fourth of July arrived, Joe called me because he was going on vacation and wanted to know his prostate-specific antigen number (which shows whether there are cancer cells present in the blood) so he could have peace of mind and enjoy his vacation with his girlfriend. The Hopkins lab was closed for the holiday, but I knew how to get hold of them, and I did. I told him the numbers; they were normal. He thanked me and I said good-bye—literally forever, or at least so I thought.

* * *

The Department of Health had a fund where money could be allocated for services, equipment, and to be donated when a medical center in need would request it. A Hasidic community in New York City needed a mammogram machine, and we donated the money for it. I felt it was necessary because many of the women married young and they needed follow-up. I talked to the rabbi and agreed to give a talk about breast cancer to the congregation, with one restriction dictated by the rabbi: I could not say the word "breast." I really wondered how I would keep my promise to him, but I had no choice—he

> "In war you can use any instrument to win it—as long as the benefits are bigger than the losses."

was standing behind the curtain that separated him from the audience and me while I was giving my talk.

I wanted to give the audience good information regarding breast cancer, and trying to keep my promise, I just grabbed my breast and started talking about the danger of "this" type of cancer. I explained how they could examine themselves and about the mammogram machine. The talk went well. The rabbi was happy, and we accomplished our goal. This kind of story demonstrates my philosophy—"In war you can use any instrument to win it—as long as the benefits are bigger than the losses" (Novello).

At the new clinic where the mammogram machine was to be placed, they implemented an idea I suggested that was relevant and compatible with their Hasidic beliefs. Every room in that building had the name of a woman from the Torah who had suffered from the disease for which women in the room were going to be treated. They wanted to name the entire clinic after me, but I asked them not to. I was afraid that their funding would disappear when I was no longer the Commissioner—such is politics.

Another win-win during my tenure was the continuation of circumcision in the Hasidic community. Tragically, one baby boy had died of herpes encephalitis after the rabbi had placed the traditional kiss at the tip of the boy's penis after the circumcision. This rite had been performed since the times of Maimonides, and it was a religious tradition. So now the Commissioner of Health—me, a Catholic Puerto Rican woman—was going to decide what would happen when herpes was not a reportable disease. Consultation occurred between the Jewish Council and me every Friday afternoon before the Sabbath for six months.

I was in awe of the Jewish Council's knowledge, their appearance, and their true dedication. So many white beards and different

Jewish head coverings. I learned to respect them, and in four hours every Friday for six months, we shaped and protected the right of Hasidic boys to be circumcised. We brought many experts to the department to help solve the stalemate, and we were successful.

This had not been easy. The Jewish Council had asked the Commissioner of Health for New York City—a Jewish doctor himself—to help them. He had refused. He felt that the death of one baby signaled the end of circumcision. And he was appalled that they came to Albany instead to see me—he didn't see the need for a Catholic woman to solve a Jewish issue.

During our time together, I realized they knew the science of circumcision but did not know how to protect the circumcised children without compromising centuries of tradition. Fortunately, a woman administrator had the book of Hasidic laws and customs translated into English as a guide for me. There I learned the science, the knowledge, and the traditions to help benefit many Jewish baby boys who could be circumcised while still protecting them from disease.

After six months of deliberations, the Jewish Council had a signed contract with New York State not to perform any circumcisions if the rabbi was infected, and the Department of Health agreed. The individuals who performed the "bris" or "brit milah" agreed to take antivirals against herpes for life—otherwise they could not perform the circumcisions. As a result of these efforts, a law was passed to make herpes a reportable disease in the state of New York approved by the New York State Public Health Council. The Commissioner of Health of New York City refused to accept the law or the process, but the circumcision of Hasidic boys as determined at the state level prevailed. It was reported in the news that a Commissioner dressed in pink had saved the circumcision of Hasidic boys. It made my day.

As I served, I had all kinds of visits from people who were Mayors or friends of the Governor or some sort of political operative who wanted me to give them licenses for nursing homes and other kinds of favors. All the hair on my body would stand up, and I'd say to myself, "I am not doing this." I never gave a permit that was not judged to be appropriate, nor a certificate of need. Never a favor to any hospital that was in the wrong. The Public Health Council weighed in. The judge advocate and peers were consulted. Never. I just didn't do favors for political gain.

Although I was the Commissioner of the Department of Health and former US Surgeon General, I was not asked to participate in the selection for the Tobacco Council for the State of New York membership, although the Governor had promised me that nothing during my tenure as Commissioner would compromise my previous job as Surgeon General. In response, I never attended a tobacco meeting, for which I blame myself. I did, however, ask each high school to assign to me two students who would become board representatives of tobacco to the state. I would meet with them in the summer, and they would tell me the things that they wanted done. Two of those students would present their efforts to the New York Senate and House of Representatives. The kids loved it and learned a lot. So did I.

At one point, I was flying back, probably from San Francisco, and I could see that my assistant was hiding the *New York Times* from me. I asked, "What is it?" and she said, "Nothing." I finally saw the article. There are shelters for the homeless and poor in New York City with laws in place to protect the inhabitants. But in some of those homes, the air conditioning was broken, and people were jumping from the roofs killing themselves in the process. The situation became very political, with people blaming me and demanding my removal as Commissioner. Upon my arrival back at my office, I gave a loud, clear, and "shrill" talk to those who had decided to speak on my behalf without my permission on such a politically life-sensitive issue. Something like that never happened again. To this day, I am very thankful to Nydia Velasquez, Congresswoman from New York City, who defended me from those who wanted me ousted.

The entire situation motivated me to study in detail each individual shelter. We changed many processes and procedures to ensure that the inhabitants were protected forever.

* * *

Joe became a full partner at the Psychiatric Institute in Washington, D.C., specializing in pediatrics, and adult and adolescent psychiatry. He wrote eight books throughout his professional life. In each one he included my name, Toni, in the acknowledgments and/or thanks, but never once did he dedicate a book to me. The book before the last one, to my surprise, he dedicated entirely to Luba, his current girlfriend. That book, published in 2001, was titled *The Myth of More: And Other Lifetraps That Sabotage the Happiness You Deserve*.

Joe had a copy of the book sent to me and to every member of my family. I read it and enjoyed the message that was central to the title. I was feeling good about his publishing success. Unbeknownst to me, Joe had removed the dedication page from each of those copies of the book.

As luck would have it, I was traveling, and my secretary at the Department of Health in Albany thought it would be a great surprise for me to have Joe's latest book, so she ordered one for me. I opened the book to thank my secretary's gesture, since she was unaware that I already had a copy. It took all my control, in front of her, to see that dedication to Luba—solely—and realize that none of the copies of the book that my family and I had received had the dedication page. Thoughtful of Joe, I guess, but very hurtful at the same time.

I did rip the dedication page out of the book that my secretary had given me. I inserted it in a letter that I wrote immediately to Joe asking him if he had forgotten something. I also pulled out of that book a paragraph on love that I thought was completely descriptive of his behavior. It described developmental disunion, where people do not learn a healthy model of married love from their parents and thus are not able to combine sex and love. I enclosed that with the letter as well. I never got a response.

* * *

Around the middle of August 2001, I went to New York City to receive a little girl from the Dominican Republic. She was going to have open heart surgery performed pro bono by the cardiac unit surgeons at NewYork-Presbyterian Hospital. Nearly a month later, on September 11, 2001, I returned to New York City for a press conference regarding the success of the little girl's open-heart surgery—to thank the hospital in the name of the Governor and the Department of Health—and to place her back on a plane to return to her hometown in the Dominican Republic.

Everything was going well. My staff and I took the train from Albany to New York City. I reviewed my remarks on the train, and we got to the station in New York City around eight a.m. My staff and I disembarked and joined my city driver who was a policewoman. Luckily, we had arrived barely minutes after the first plane hit the first World Trade Center tower. Otherwise, we would have been stuck in the train tunnel.

As sirens starting wailing, our driver mentioned the news was reporting that maybe a small weather plane had collided with one of the World Trade Center towers. We got in the car and started driving toward NewYork-Presbyterian Hospital where we were to meet all the rest of the entourage for the press conference. On our way, we saw maybe seventeen ambulances driving at full speed—all going together—toward the World Trade Center area. We turned on the radio.

It was a Tuesday morning, a beautiful fall day in New York City. Crisp, comfortable, and clear. It was supposed to be the day of the primaries to elect the next mayor. As it unfolded, the primaries were canceled because of the terrorist attack on the World Trade Center towers.

As we were driving to NewYork-Presbyterian, I got a call. We were to go to the fourteenth floor of what is now called the Irving Pavilion of NewYork-Presbyterian and wait. The press conference had been canceled.

To this day, I do not know what happened to the little girl who had heart surgery. Hopefully, she made it home safely. I also realized that most of the seventeen ambulances never came back to the hospital ER. The noises were maddening, the people chaotic, remembering that something similar had happened in the towers a few years before and there was not much damage. This time, however, was different.

My staff and I arrived at the fourteenth floor, where the office of the NewYork-Presbyterian President was, and through the glass windows I saw the second plane hit the second tower. We also watched the collapse of both towers and the smoke. It looked like the movie *The Fog*, and to me it felt like the beginning of a third World War. With the collapse of the towers, all antennae on the towers were destroyed, and standard communication channels were no longer working.

Even though I was surrounded by people, I felt scared, shaky, and alone. Like everyone else, I just wanted to go home. Suddenly, it hit me—New York City was in chaos. I was the Health Commissioner of the State. There was work to be done. Stop feeling scared—and get going!

It's almost like when someone has a heart attack, their heart has momentarily stopped, but they need you to resuscitate them back to life. You do not think of anything else and in spite of your fears, you just keep going and doing the things that need to be done to get that person to live again.

I felt like that at that moment, and I went into action. Where do I start? What do I need to do? A call came in on a walkie talkie—the Governor was requesting us to go back to Albany and institute the disaster and recovery plan. We were to go to the basement level of the Police Academy in Albany—the bunker as it was called—where there were endless computers, screens, and cubicles, all of them monitoring areas in the city. From there we could guide whatever was necessary—beds, personnel, blood, equipment, and so forth—wherever it was needed. What we couldn't do from there was to save the thousands of people killed that day from this horrendous catastrophe.

On that fateful day as we watched the smoke and debris, we communicated on shortwave radios. My policewoman driver picked me up, and we left for Albany and the bunker. Minutes after we left, all entrances to the city were closed. If we had been delayed by just five minutes, we would not have been able to leave. The airport was closed. The bridges were closed. The city was closed.

It is important to mention here that when the previous incident occurred at the World Trade Center towers (in 1993), it was discovered that radio channels for both the police and firefighters had deficits. The former had fixed their radio frequency but apparently not the latter. This probably explains why, when the towers collapsed, the police got the calls to leave the area but the firefighters did not—they kept climbing the stairways. That day was the deadliest day in the life of a firefighter.

After establishing the bunker, I returned to New York City. I was able to return as my driver was a policewoman with a white shirt, and she said they wouldn't keep her out. I was more needed in the city than in the bunker. I visited every hospital in the areas close to the towers to follow up with the victims who had survived. There were not many. Every hospital was on high alert. I was checking on the hospitals, the blood supply, and the medical personnel. When I went to the hospitals, I told every administrator that no one was to be asked about health insurance. Then I went to the city morgue and to the burn unit of NewYork-Presbyterian. The morgue had run out of body bags to carry the dead. In some there were fingers; in others there were bodies. Some body bags had only arms or legs—whatever was left of a human found in the debris.

I called the military, and they sent me as many body bags as we needed during the crisis. Similarly, the burn unit at New York-Presbyterian was full, and they needed help, especially since the mortality rate increases significantly in people whose bodies are more than 40 percent burned—even in the highly specialized units. I requested burn nurses from the military units in San Antonio to come and help—and they came. In addition, I made a plea for every expert in mental health to make themselves available for the mental health crisis that was evolving. I really believe that having been Surgeon General before Commissioner and knowing the Surgeons General of the other services helped a lot.

Over the ensuing days, many actions needed to be taken by many people. There was no budget for the state to handle this sort of crisis, so the Governor got both state congressional chambers together, and they were able to pass an emergency budget.

Another issue that needed to be handled was the identification of body parts that could only be done with DNA. But the only DNA available in New York State was DNA in police precincts. When the Governor requested that we find alternatives, I remembered then that the former Director of the NIH Cancer Institute had left his post and was now in charge of a company that traced DNA. I called him and with his company's help, we were able to trace as many as eight hundred samples per day, allowing us to start identifying people who up to that point had only been pictures displayed on walls.

Another worrisome issue: the wall that separated the island of Manhattan from the Hudson River was being pummeled constantly with debris that had been deposited in the river when the towers collapsed. Would it hold? There were so many explosions daily. What would happen if that wall broke and the river came in? We also knew that two weeks before 9/11 the air-conditioning system at the World Trade Center had received a new infusion of freon. And there were around two thousand cars in the parking area of the lower parts of the towers with gasoline in their tanks. In addition, on the third floor of one of the towers was ammunition, guns and grenades for the Coast Guard. Issues appeared regularly. How many trains could be run? How many tunnels were disabled? What emergencies were happening at the hospitals? Some of these issues we kept to ourselves—we didn't want to tell the press because then the public would worry to no good end. But we prepared for the consequences of every one of these.

We had to set boundaries associated with the cleanup and the tragedy itself. When debris was sent to the landfill area, we requested the news outlets be more respectful regarding the visits and the images. When children started drawing jumpers, we requested more respect regarding how this was affecting the children, and the news media complied.

Families came with pictures of loved ones asking if anyone had seen them. This was incredibly heartbreaking. The Governor and Mayor Rudy Giuliani opened areas where volunteers could get all the necessary information to trace in any manner possible the loved ones who were still missing. In addition, the Governor facilitated widows' and widowers' ability to withdraw money out of bank accounts, even though no dead person had been identified. This was the first time this had happened, and it helped relieve the worries of the survivors.

Smells started coming from the debris of the towers. Rat traps were placed around the site. But the smells were coming from rotten food left on stoves, in open refrigerators, and on tables, when people started running. Thank goodness, we had one less problem to deal with from a health perspective—no rats.

Three months later, the last fire in the tower area was finally squelched, and the wall had held. Up to that time, every day from one to two p.m. there would be a meeting in the area of Mayor Giuliani's office where the Governor, the Secretary of State, the Director of Emergencies, the Director of Police and Firemen, and I would meet and discuss every single item pertinent to the towers and the surrounding tunnels, hospitals, and subways.

All the public health topics I had read in my textbooks were put to use during and after September 11. I felt very proud during those

> **"Facts always. Never opinions in emergencies."**

three months. The media would pause after the Governor spoke—to give space to the Hispanic media to hear it in Spanish from me. I received the biggest award that the National Governors Association can give for my performance during September 11. I am still in awe that someone was following what I was doing—when actually all I did was what was expected of the Health Commissioner of the state. I have used the knowledge I gained during that time to help people in other emergencies, because emergencies keep coming! For example, I used that knowledge in Puerto Rico after Hurricane Maria, during the January 2020 earthquake, and with COVID-19. I don't know everything, but I will search for the answers to the things I don't know. Facts always. Never opinions in emergencies.

One regret I have, though, is that during those months that I was in New York City dealing with 9/11, my deputy was back in Albany running the department. He was not able to come to the city to see it with his own eyes. I wish he could have seen the devastation firsthand.

* * *

In November 2001, I was scheduled on a nine a.m. flight out of JFK to Puerto Rico. The next gate over from ours was very busy—it was an 8 a.m. flight destined for Santo Domingo, Dominican Republic. The flight had been delayed. We boarded our flight to Puerto Rico, our plane took off, but almost immediately the pilot came on the intercom and said, "I'm sorry, we have to return to the airport." As we were landing, my niece from Puerto Rico called and left a voicemail. She is always there when something bad happens to me and her message was, "Titi, if you are alive, please call me. I am praying that you were not on the flight that crashed." We landed. We had no idea what had happened. Every plane flying out of a New York area airport had been ground stopped. All the luggage was piled on the tarmac—meaning that there were literally thousands of black suitcases. We could see smoke somewhere on the horizon, but no one had yet told us what had happened. After we landed, I called my niece and told her that I was okay. My driver at the time was again the policewoman, a no-nonsense woman, tough. She saw us looking for our luggage on the tarmac and said, "Oh, my God. Oh, my God." Then she said, "This is the first time in my life that I need someone to hug me." So we hugged her, even though my assistant and I could also have used a hug and support. The plane that crashed was American Airlines Flight 587 and the date was November 12, 2001, not long after the events of 9/11. Everyone aboard the plane died.

The next flight I took was with Governor Pataki. He felt it was important to visit the Dominican Republic and pay our respects to the people who had died in the crash of American Airlines Flight 587. We wanted to give our condolences to the President of the Dominican Republic and find out how we could help. Most of the people who died had been Dominican residents of the United States. Before we got off the plane, the Governor reminded us that no one was to accept any gift with a value beyond $75, because that was illegal. The man who was receiving us in Santo Domingo and who had made the condolences flight possible had political connections. As soon as we entered the office of the president of the Dominican Republic, he presented the Governor with a painting from one of the famous Dominican painters. Of course, its value must have been more than $75. There was no politically acceptable way for the Governor to refuse the gift or the painting.

From the Dominican Republic, the entourage went to Puerto Rico. It was election time, and the Puerto Rican Governor was helping the New York Governor in the election race and vice versa. There was a wonderful state dinner in San Juan that we all attended.

These trips reminded me that in difficult moments, you have to forget that you are busy, and you have to do what's right. It's like when employees come and tell me, "Dr. Novello, you are eating, and people come, and they want a picture, and they want an autograph." You always take the picture and sign the autograph. You don't say, "Excuse me, I'm having dinner. Please come back later." You want their first impression to be favorable. Even if I'm tired or hungry, I put that aside and try to be as sociable as I can. This attitude has helped me through life, but it has not been easy. First impressions can be crucial in your job acceptance when you are in politics.

* * *

In 2002, I learned from Joe's sister that Dad Novello had died. It was on Joe's birthday, and he had been visiting his family. His father had a heart attack and Joe had administered CPR, but Dad did not survive. I went to the funeral in Ohio as I thought it was the right thing to do. Joe and I hadn't spoken since his prostate surgery. Mom Novello was happy to see me, but it was very difficult sitting in the same hearse with Joe and Luba, his girlfriend. It was rainy, chilly, and cold. All of a sudden, Joe came over and put his coat around my shoulders. Maybe he appreciated that I came to his father's funeral from Puerto Rico where it was hot. I came because I really cared for them. I had been their daughter-in-law for twenty-four years.

On New Year's Day, 2004, Mom Novello called to tell me that Joe had given Luba an engagement ring while they were on a Caribbean cruise. That day, I left my hometown in Puerto Rico to go to the airport for the afternoon flight to Washington instead of the six p.m. flight I usually took. When I got to the American Airlines window, the

American Club concierge was doing the check-in behind the reservation counter. She called me and said, "Let me help you—I haven't seen you in a while." She checked her computer and told me what awful seats they had given me and my husband. I froze, never imagining that Joe would be on the same plane. I asked if our friend Luba was on the plane as well. And the woman replied, "Yes, the three of you are in 14A, 14B, and 14C."

I asked the American Airlines concierge if there was a first-class seat as I was petrified of sitting next to the newly engaged couple for three hours. She said, "No, sorry." I was teary and confused, and she looked at me and said, "Is everything okay?" To my surprise, I started crying (I rarely cry except at sad movies), and I explained that I had gotten divorced (which no one in Puerto Rico knew) and that my ex and his new fiancée were the ones sitting close to me!

She understood immediately and said, "I don't know who I'm going to bump from first class—but you are going in first class." And so I did! When Joe and Luba were boarding, they didn't see me—but she kept flashing her new engagement ring for everyone to see. I knew the flight attendant after so many flights to and from Puerto Rico and asked her if they still carried champagne aboard. When she replied affirmatively, I asked her to take two glasses to the newly engaged couple sitting in Row 14. They declined. I had seen Joe in the boarding area while Luba had gone to the ladies' room. I shocked him to death when I tapped him on the shoulder and congratulated him. He had forgotten that I always traveled back to the States from Puerto Rico on New Year's Day. When we got to Dulles, he came toward me and asked me if my family had liked the Christmas presents he sent. I said they had, and we chit-chatted while Luba was up against the wall moving her feet and face in dismay.

I think that Joe was naive and didn't think he was going to have to marry Luba immediately. Knowing him, I thought the ring could be a form of "layaway" for the time being. However, when they arrived in her hometown, they discovered that one week after the engagement, her brother (unbeknownst to Joe) had reserved the Country Club for a wedding in June. So they got married.

During the years I lived in Albany, I would fly to Ohio whenever Mom Novello got sick. I was almost her caretaker. When the Pope came to Ohio, I flew there because I knew Mom would want to watch that on television, and I stayed with her while she watched it. She also loved baseball, so we would watch baseball together. When Mom died, I was the one holding the picture of the family in front of her because she wanted to see her family for the last time. So in the end, I was very close to my mother-in-law and father-in-law. Before he died, I would send goodies to Dad Novello every week because Mom was in a nursing home, and I knew he was alone. He used to call me *bambola,* which means "doll" in Italian. That was quite a compliment, since in the beginning he was not happy that Joe was marrying a Puerto Rican. At the end, he cared very deeply for me, and I for him.

* * *

A doctor colleague of mine had a wife with advanced breast cancer, and she was in hospice. I was getting ready to go to Paris, France, to attend an AIDS conference, but I wanted to pay my respects before I left. I knew that if she was in a coma when I went to visit her before my trip, she might not be alive when I came back. I went to visit, and, as I suspected, she was in a coma. I asked my colleague what his plans were. He said, "Well, last week we moved to the house that she always wanted, and now she will not see it. All of the boxes are still there, and we haven't done any of the unpacking because this happened. I don't want the grandchildren to see her in a coma, I want them to remember her the way she was." And as I was standing by her bed, words came out of me—I have no idea where they came from. I said, "You know what? She's going to get out of this coma, she's going to ask for something hot to drink, you're going to take her home, you're going to unpack all your boxes, and then when you show her the grandchildren, she's going to go then."

I got back from Paris and my doorbell rang. It was the doctor. He said, "You are a witch." I said, "A what?" He said, "You are a witch." I said, "What in the world happened?" He said that after I left, his wife opened her eyes. She asked for something hot to drink. They went home. They unpacked all the boxes. She got the house arranged the way she wanted. She spoke with her grandchildren and then she passed. My God, I still wonder—where did my thinking come from?

* * *

While I was working in Albany, New York, I got a call from the mayor of my hometown, Fajardo, Puerto Rico. He was a friend of the family and perhaps even one of the thousands of students who had passed through Mami's classroom during her almost sixty-nine years of educational service. He invited me to present her accomplishments to the Fajardo Assembly as they were considering naming a school after her that was about to be built. It would be the largest one in eastern Puerto Rico. I was very pleased and ready to present what was needed to make this a reality. I assumed that most of the assembly members knew Mami, that most of them had been her pupil at one point, and that really her accomplishments were already known.

The theme of my presentation was differentiating between a teacher and a true educator. Mami was in the latter group. I thought everything was going well. I had flown in just for the presentation and planned to fly back to Albany the next afternoon. I decided to call the mayor and thank him for his invitation. To my shock and surprise, he said that Mami's nomination had been sent to a committee rather than it being approved on the spot—as he had assured me previously would be the case. I asked to speak with the Chairman of the assembly. To my surprise, I recognized him as the new principal of the Catholic school, but I also remembered him as a student who had not been enamored with my mother's classroom techniques.

The Chairman, very cocky, told me that the assembly had decided to name the school after a teacher who lived in the area, who had taught industrial arts for many years, and who was missing a leg—he had a prosthesis. I was even more confused. I told him that I knew when things go into committee that is a nice way of letting them die a slow death. He agreed and assumed that the conversation had ended, and the matter was decided. I remember asking him, "Why are you playing politics with something so important for my mother?" He was cold and distant. I told him if he played politics, I was about to play bigger politics.

I rescheduled my flight and instead of returning to Albany I went to the capital city of San Juan and went straight to the Office of the Speaker of the House. I explained my case. His response was something on the order of: "When the Big Assembly speaks, the little one obeys." Needless to say, the school was named after my mother.

I also came to realize that at that time, the mayor had a political battle to win in the neighborhood where the school was being built. Thus, naming the school for the industrial arts teacher instead of my mother—who had been the principal of the only junior high in town for the last forty-four years—would not have been a win-win for him.

The day of the building's dedication in December of 2005, Mami was very sick. She had just fallen and fractured three ribs. After much convincing, I told her, if need be, I would be proud and happy to speak for her as long as she would attend. She agreed then to dress and come to the dedication ceremony. At the front of the school that day were some protestors with signs. There were not many, but they were there. Mami was sad and in physical pain.

Unbeknownst to the protestors and because Mami had always been a very good friend of the policemen in my hometown, I invited the police band from San Juan to perform at the dedication. They came in two loaded school buses—in uniform and with their instruments in their hands in black bags. When the protestors saw the policemen—which they assumed was a SWAT team—they ran away.

The audience at the ceremony was a who's who of leading educators and dignitaries from Fajardo, including the Mayor. I gave a speech in which I requested that although the school carried Mami's name—Ana Delia Flores—that the amphitheater be named after the industrial arts teacher. The audience loved the suggestion and applauded. Mami was happy. Finally, she was receiving the recognition that she deserved for her sixty-nine years of service to the education system of Puerto Rico.

* * *

In 2005, an empty hospital bed cost the state of New York about $22,000 per year. Governor Pataki decided that, until further decisions could be made about the economics of hospital operation, any hospital with empty beds might have to be closed, with only the ERs staying open. A committee was created, and I was not asked to participate on this study committee; my deputy and my Chief of Press were the designated representatives.

The committee progressed with its efforts in parallel to the 2006 elections in which Eliot Spitzer became Governor, and the administration of the state of New York switched from Republican to Democrat after twelve years of a Republican administration. I had come across important information that maybe the Chief of Press could have used inside information to enhance his career and could have provided advance knowledge to groups that might be subject to closure before the Governor was given or acted on the report.

I went to report what I thought was happening to the Chief of Operations of the Governor—and told him I was intending to report this behavior to the FBI. I was told not to contact the FBI. He suggested it could open a Pandora's Box, but instead I was given the okay to fire the Chief of Press. From that day forward, every single moment of my public life was bad press and bad publicity.

When Governor Pataki's term was nearing its end in 2006, and I assumed I would be replaced as Commissioner, I began to look for other jobs. I got a call from Governor Jeb Bush of Florida's Chief of Staff. His Secretary of Health had left for another opportunity. Governor Bush said he wanted the best—and his Chief of Staff contacted me. I said to Bush's Chief of Staff, "Look, Bush is Republican. Pataki is Republican. This is the last year in both of their terms." We were having a bad epidemic of SARS, and I felt I couldn't leave Governor Pataki to go work in Florida for one year. I knew I could have done a good job, but I didn't want to leave a job I had had for almost six years. Loyalty is very important to me.

I did some interviews during that time. My first interview was for a job to be President of one of the medical schools in Pennsylvania. When the interview was finished, the person who had brought me in for the interview said the job was mine. However, in the end, with a new President coming to the university system, the job went to someone who was already employed at the medical school.

Then the University of Michigan called me. Somebody had put in my name for a new executive health affairs position for the University. I was so touched to hear from my alma mater. I interviewed with the board. Afterward, I got a call from the Chairman of the Board informing me that I had been selected to be the Executive Vice President of Health Affairs at the University of Michigan. It would have been a very exciting time to be in Michigan—the Governor was a woman, and the President of the university was a woman. But then the President's assistant called me to say that the President was rescinding the offer. She said she felt more comfortable with the former Dean she had had at the University of Iowa, and she wanted to offer the job to him. So I accepted the new President's wishes.

Perhaps I should have called the Chairman of the Board for an explanation—but my pride took over and I didn't.

That was the last time that I competed for any job in academia. They did later ask me to apply to be the Dean of the School of Public Health at the University of Michigan, but I declined. Not good enough for one—not good enough for the second.

I was hired eventually by the Florida Children's Hospital and started my work there as Vice President, Women and Children, in August of 2008.

It is customary for each New York Health Commissioner to have a portrait commissioned to hang on a department wall. My portrait was going to be more expensive than the previous Commissioners', and this made the news media. Almost all the other portraits of the Commissioners were painted by the wife of one of them, and the last one, almost seven years before, cost $8,000. I told the artist I was using that I needed to keep the cost below what he was planning to charge, and he agreed to the price that I suggested: $10,000. The portrait was unveiled shortly before my departure. At the unveiling I said to my employees, tell me if you think this is an accurate portrait. They gave me a standing ovation. In the portrait, I was standing near the flags of the United States, New York State, and the USPHS and wearing a pin in honor of my mother. Mami always wore flowers on her lapel, so I always wore a broach remembering her commitment. This time, it had the US Public Health Service emblem.

One's retirement party is supposed to be an enjoyable event where your accomplishments are celebrated. My deputy came very late to my retirement party, handed me a plaque, gave a lame, pedestrian speech, and left. That morning he had been appointed as Chief of Operations for Governor Spitzer. He had served for more than six years as my deputy and for four years as deputy to the previous Commissioner and Governor Pataki. Life is full of surprises. Job security over loyalty.

CHAPTER 9

Framed by the Albany 5

The Inspector General of the state of New York sent me a letter around October 2008 requesting my presence in Albany. I had just started my job at the Florida Hospital in August when the letter arrived at my office. My secretary delivered it to me with a snicker on his face—I knew there was going to be trouble. Even religious hospitals have gossip.

I could not think why the Inspector General was contacting me. I decided to get in touch with the lawyer who had been in charge of the legal office of the Health Commissioner. He served with me and knew me well for three or four years. He told me that he could not help me because he had been special assistant for Attorney General Spitzer, and that it would be a conflict of interest for him. He recommended, however, that I should never go to a meeting with or respond to a letter from the Inspector General unless I was accompanied by legal counsel.

I followed his advice and contacted the only law firm I knew at the time, the one that had helped me obtain my divorce in 1994. Now, it was October 2008. They took the case, charging $500 per hour. I only heard from the assigned lawyer when I called, and I was never told by him or anyone else what the issue was behind the Inspector General's request to visit Albany. It was probably late October or early November when the attorney told me that it might be an issue with my driver or my car during the time I was Commissioner and that the District Attorney in New York was interested in pursuing my case. No more was said, found, or reported to me.

I heard again from that attorney a week or so before Christmas when he told me that he didn't have a license to practice in New York and thus could not help me anymore. He dropped me like a hot tamale. I went crazy. So little time before Christmas, a case with the Inspector General, no information offered regarding the reasons why I was in trouble, and I didn't know what to do! I felt there must be something wrong when eventually the law firm, without my asking, returned the $5,000 retainer. I was even more confused—did they know something I didn't?

And then I remembered another attorney. I had met him when we both sat on the board of a cancer prevention nonprofit—we met through his wife who had died of ovarian cancer. I called him a week before Christmas and explained my case. He said, "Commissioner, it's Christmas. I'll take you because I know you. I'll investigate." He was kind, thoughtful, and took my case—perhaps in memory of his wife, or perhaps it was because I sounded so lost and dejected that he decided to take what appeared to be a losing case. But he was one of the top twenty-five lawyers in the state at the time, and he honored his oath and his reputation and took the challenge.

It was maybe the first week in January that he contacted me and said, "Commissioner, it's too late. The report of your case has been written and submitted." I thought, *Oh, my God. What now?*

I screamed. How could my case have been written when I didn't even know the reasons I was summoned? He told me that the kinds of things he found in my case are things that lawyers discuss in their offices. It should not have gotten to this level. One of the charges involved me requiring my staff to water my plants. My plants were all silk. Then, as a very knowledgeable lawyer, he said that he would never allow me to testify before a grand jury, since in cases like this, they might come up with things that could be worse than expected, and he did not think that I could get a fair hearing.

My niece in Puerto Rico called me the morning of January 26, 2009. According to the front page of the *New York Times*, I was being accused of multiple counts, including felonies, and faced probable jail time. That was how I learned for the first time about the charges against me—I read them in the *New York Times*! I immediately called the woman who had been my Chief of Staff while I was Commissioner. She was my friend, and she knew me well. Perhaps she knew something I didn't. I said, "What is going on? Did you read this?" She said, "Commissioner, I have been told I cannot speak to you." I said, "Oh, my God, you are part of the prosecution," and I hung up. I was dumbfounded, confused, and felt betrayed by the system—and more so by my Chief of Staff of four years, my trusted ally!

This was the same day of the first research lecture I was in charge of at the Florida Hospital. The topic was obesity, and the presenter was from the CDC. As I walked into my boss's office to get ready for the speaker's arrival, my boss said to me, "You have to take a leave of absence." I asked how they could judge me before the court had judged me. Human Resources then asked me to take a two-week leave of absence while they processed the news and ramifications of this event. During that time, reporters were outside of my house. Those two weeks were hell. I didn't leave my house the entire time—I don't even think I ate because I couldn't go to the supermarket. The press were everywhere.

I remember vividly the moment I went back to Albany. It was the first time I knew the substance of the accusations against me. Before I had only known what I had read in the *New York Times*. I had always loved Albany, its people, the Midwest flavor of decency of the area residents, the congeniality of those I worked with, and the feeling of accomplishment from working in the department.

All those images went blank as I walked through the Albany airport and saw all the television screens—right on top of my head was my image and name on those screens, declaring me a possible felon.

I wanted to die, hide, cry, disappear. I felt naked, as if I had been raped. But still I managed to get to my lawyer's office for our first appointment.

My attorney told me I could not get a fair trial in Albany because the person who accused me was Black, and so was the District Attorney, his deputy, and the Governor. He then said that my case was an Administrative Processing Offense. But, he said, because of how far the case had progressed, we would need to plead the case. This was because he saw no other alternative and because jail time was part of the case.

It was at this time that my mother had a heart attack. I felt the time had come to close the chapter. Thus, I went along with the attorney's recommendation, and I decided to do whatever was necessary—my mother's life was more important than me, the case, or the charges against me. The stress was also getting to me—I was now down to 118 pounds; my normal weight was around 140 pounds.

The first meeting with the District Attorney was supposed to be private according to my attorney. I could not believe how many cameras and reporters were waiting for my arrival at the courthouse. Somebody wanted me noticed or needed me to have more punishment than he or she had already personally inflicted. I went into the office with the Assistant District Attorney and my lawyer. For the first time, I was told of the accusations that should have been explained to me from the beginning by my first lawyer. The one I remember most shockingly was an allegation that I had signed false documents regarding my driver's working times and overtime pay. In my mind, I never submitted this information—the driver was doing that, not me. I also recalled a lot of new forms brought by my secretary that I started signing toward the end of my tenure as Commissioner.

I responded that I used to sign close to a hundred pieces of paper a day. The important ones I signed with my full name. The routine papers I signed with a very short and convoluted version of my name.

The Assistant District Attorney said she didn't care. Looking straight in my face, she told me she didn't want any explanation. I repeated my reasons why the case against me might be wrong. She said she believed my driver more than she believed me. My lawyer looked at me—and we both realized that her opinions against me, albeit wrong, were too strong to be overturned or explained. So we left the office confused, somewhat flabbergasted, but more than anything—shocked. And angry. I was and had been framed, and there was no way out.

We didn't talk to the press. My lawyer would not allow me to when we left the District Attorney's office for the first time.

My second trip back to Albany was for the sentencing. I was told not to wear anything flashy—instead, conservative clothing, no large jewelry, normal hair, and so forth. I really didn't have to be asked because that was my modus operandi anyway.

That morning, the courtroom was full, including reporters from Puerto Rico. My lawyer and I were called to the front—and then came the surprises. The judge praised my work as Commissioner for about five to seven minutes, during which I became hopeful that things would turn out better for my side. Then he proceeded to blast out the most painful words I have ever heard: "You stand here now as a convicted felon." He then proceeded to call me arrogant and entitled, abusive to staff, and that all along I knew I was violating the law but did it anyway. All of the words were so similar to what I had heard previously from the Assistant District Attorney, and she was standing right next to the judge.

I couldn't remove my eyes from the judge's face, afraid that he might treat me worse. All the time, my lawyer is saying under his breath, "What the hell is this?"

We left the court, and this time my lawyer let me speak to the press. The members of the press were my friends. And the press was saying to each other, "Leave her alone. Can't you see she's upset?"

I said something to the effect that in spite of this episode, I was not going to lose trust in either humankind or government but that I was very sad for those who accused me because they were the ones I had trusted the most. I couldn't believe that they would want to destroy me and my legacy because I didn't give them the jobs that they wanted after I was no longer in charge. I wished them well and then I left. I also said someday they will not be able to look me in the eye—but I will be able to look into theirs.

The punishment was restitution of $22,500, a fine of $5,000, and 250 hours of community service at an Albany health clinic. I did not have that money and I went to Mami—she took all that she had saved in the teacher's association and gave me the money to pay the restitution and fine. After the sentencing, I did the cheek swab for the DNA testing and had pictures taken of my face and side. It was very sad to see the same policemen that cared for me placing me in front of the camera, swabbing my mouth. They seemed as embarrassed as I was, and I dare to say that some of their eyes were as wet as mine. I then left with my attorney. During the settlement negotiations, he had ensured that I still had my passport and my right to vote. This was possible because there were never any bribes—either giving or receiving. In addition, my medical license in New York was never at risk, so I still have it and pay my dues. There was never a certificate of need, or a licensing with favors given, nor money ever accepted. Thus, I can always feel proud that my felony was done to humble and humiliate me in front of my peers. Like my lawyer had suggested—this type of complaint is generally resolved in lawyers' offices, not in court. But we were never given the chance.

I decided to serve all 250 hours of community service at one time. I volunteered at the Koinonia Primary Care Clinic in West Hill for the poor and needy run by Dr. Bob Paeglow. He was a great humanitarian doctor in the poorest section of town where some of his patients were drug users and/or unhoused. He

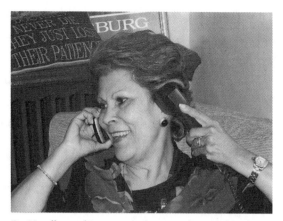

Dr. Novello speaking on two phones as she completes her community service at the Koinonia Primary Care Clinic.

oversaw me during my sentence. I decided to stay in the upstairs rooms where some of the clinics' patients lived and did my 250 hours—two months—every day. I opened the clinic. I closed the clinic. I washed the dishes, made the coffee, emptied the garbage, swept the floors, made appointments, drew blood, and gave advice to whomever needed it. I requested equipment from friends to equip the clinic and it was given. I learned of the need of those that by no fault of their own are not as lucky as the rest of us. I really respected my time there and lived in one little room with everyone there. I worked from about eight a.m. until about eight p.m. every day.

Throughout the ordeal and later, I heard from several people who said that they had been called by the District Attorney's office of New York about everything I had done in the past year. The office was fishing and had found nothing that would make me a felon. To this day, I do not know if any of them were reelected to their political posts. I don't really care. Someone said it best—"Karma never forgets your address."

I have never been back to Albany.

Hindsight is always good but comes too late. I was not a New Yorker; I was an outsider to New York politics, a naive Puerto Rican. I didn't play their games, and I didn't grant favors. I wasn't playing "politics." When Spitzer became governor, his team wanted blood, a scapegoat. And I was no longer there to defend myself. They had spent too much time, too much money, and had found nothing major. Spitzer had a reputation that he would not let you go unless and until you were found guilty. When Spitzer and his team arrived in Albany, the first victim was me—the first and only person to be put on the chopping block.

I remembered that my secretary started giving me all these papers to sign—and passed them very fast as I signed them without being able to read them. About two to three months before the new Governor came in, the new Chief of Staff stopped accompanying me to places. My previous Chief of Staff had always accompanied me to these places before. My pictures in the *New York Post* became the ugliest I had ever seen—since I had fired the Chief of Press.

My attorney told me that there were five accusers—I call them the "Albany 5"—and that there were five depositions. He only wanted me to read one—the one from my Chief of Staff. I asked, "If there are five depositions, why do you want me to read that one?" And he said he remembered that I had said that if I ever had a daughter, I wanted her to be like my Chief of Staff. What an eye opener—a Judas or Brutus in my life. I was in shock, in pain, in tears.

When I read her statement, it was shocking. She said she never told me what to do. That she accompanied me only a minimal number of times. God knows that my whole agenda was in her hands for four years and nothing moved in my life unless it passed her approval. Until I read her deposition, I believed that the other four accusers were the bad ones (my deputy, my new acting Chief of Staff, my driver, and my secretary). I could never have fathomed that my Chief of Staff would have double-crossed me the way she did! She just threw me to the wolves.

In hindsight, it appears that I alienated several individuals within the department—enough so that they would frame me and put me up on charges. How might that have happened? Here are some of my thoughts.

About a month after my arrival in Albany, a person in charge of finances from the office of the Governor was brought to my office with a person wanting a certificate of need for a nursing home. He was a friend of the Governor and probably a donor. I was surprised at this request as I had not been briefed about the nursing home, and I got concerned because the Chief of Hospital Services was not present at the meeting. It gave me the feeling that the donor was flaunting his relationship with the Governor, and that I was an easy target for giving the certificate of need. I thanked him for his visit and denied his certificate. One possible strike against me.

I discovered almost six months into the job that one of the most liked members of the department's hospital team was married to a consultant in a very powerful law firm. That consultant—as luck would have it, was performing the legal work for almost all the certificates of need approved from the Department of Health. I started looking into this. I even spoke to the Chief of Hospital Services to ask how he felt about this. I had begun to understand how close the relationships were in the department, and this group had one of the closest relationships of all. They wanted to protect the employee from being sanctioned—or worse, fired. I spoke to the employee and asked if his wife, who worked for the law firm, was an employee, a consultant, or pro bono. I found that she was being rewarded very handsomely for what appeared to be pro bono services. I informed him that there was a significant conflict of interest here and one of them would have to stop. He said his wife's salary was important to their livelihood and thus she would have to stay in her job. He decided to retire from the department. It was a very sad day. His friends were not pleased with my decision. They wanted me to look the other way, but I could not, so I rode out the storm. Strike two perhaps?

In addition, I learned from reading magazines and newspapers that my Deputy Commissioner had received quite a few presents from the Jewish community—tickets to ball games, ties, cookware, and so on. He admitted receiving the gifts and promised to return them. Since his gift receiving had already made the news, I had to do something, and therefore I reduced his pay for two weeks and reported how we solved it. I don't think the Deputy Commissioner ever forgave me. His father had been the Commissioner of the Department of Health. Now, the deputy's reputation was somewhat tainted. He was a ticking bomb, ready to explode. That probably explains why during my retirement party his comments were short, unemotional, and pedestrian—and he was late to the event. He eventually rose to positions of authority within the department under Governor Spitzer after working for Governor Pataki for two of his three terms. Srike three?

At one time, I thought I would be given a pardon by Governor David Paterson who understood that I had been entrapped. I was told by the Secretary of State at the time that Governor Paterson would consider pardoning me. I got everything in order—the request, the letters of recommendation, and I sent them. Unbeknownst to me, the deadline had been October 31. My request arrived in November, and it was rejected for not meeting the submission date. I buried the disappointment and continued working.

CHAPTER 10

Duty Still Calls

I will always be thankful for Florida Hospital. Despite the charges against me in New York, they never pulled the rug out from under my feet. They did not fire me. They did require that I take a leave of absence after the charges were made public in the *New York Times*, and after my conviction they changed my title and responsibilities. Instead of being the Vice President of Women and Children of the Children's Hospital I was named the Executive Director for Public Policy. I stayed in that role until I retired in 2014. I will be forever grateful.

Once I was in Florida, I became aware of the Don Quixote Prize—a very prestigious prize in Orlando, awarded by the Hispanic Chamber of Commerce. I received a notice that they were going to consider me for a prize in one of the categories. I asked one of my work colleagues about such a nomination and she said to wait a year. I debated my response and sent in my information anyway. I wanted to know my standing in the community, if any.

A couple of months went by, and I got a call from the President of the Hispanic Chamber of Commerce. He said I had been selected for the Lifetime Achievement Award. There was a video introduction for me in which Supreme Court Justice Sandra Day O'Connor appeared and said hello to her friend, Toni. The audience was very pleased with her words of praise, and I was, more than ever, very proud of her. I was given ten minutes to speak, and it appeared that I brought down the house—standing ovation, tears, screams, everything. I did not know that they had requested Justice Sonia Sotomayor to say a few words. She did not. I was thus so thankful for the comments of Justice O'Connor.

* * *

When Mami's health began to decline, she could no longer live independently. I am very grateful that I was able to care for her in her final years.

As I said, Mami had a heart attack in Puerto Rico in early 2009, when all the issues caused by the Albany 5 were happening. The press in Puerto Rico started circling her for information. She was very sad as she knew my reputation would be tainted. My brother, Tomas, who lived in a gated community, took her home with him.

Then for a time, we shuttled her between my home in Orlando and Tomas's home in Puerto Rico. She spent three months with me and then one month with Tomas. Eventually, his retirement business needed all of his attention, so I took charge of her health. She stayed with me until she died.

At Christmastime 2009, I took Mami to Puerto Rico and invited all her friends to see her at her house. She was happy. It was the last time that she saw her own house. It was always a dream of hers to have a house on a corner, with big balconies and a great bedroom displaying all her awards. That is exactly what she got in Orlando with me. And she was happy.

While I worked at Florida Hospital, I hired help for her that came every weekday from eight a.m. to four p.m. I never took Mami to see my new office, however. It did not compare to former offices of mine that she had seen—both as Surgeon General and Commissioner of Health of the State of New York. I didn't want her to compare or to show disappointment.

Mami was afraid of the dark by herself in my house, so I slept with her. This continued even after she had a stroke. After her stroke, she would wake me up—she would be planning the first day of school. She would be calling her vice principal, asking, "Did you check this room? Did you get the books? Get me the children right now to tell them exactly what the expectations are for their uniforms and how they need to look." She was doing all of this in her sleep, but it did not allow me to sleep in peace. Somehow we managed.

Mami developed chronic renal failure after her stroke. However, she did not want dialysis after seeing her sister die at Bethesda Naval Hospital; Tomas's wife had also had dialysis for multiple myeloma with kidney failure. I never pushed her to get dialysis. As a nephrologist, I kept her diet low in potassium and liquid and tried to give her the best quality of life that I could. She developed a condition called open hydrocephalus, a buildup of fluids in cavities within the brain. The hospital where I worked had a new research method to treat this condition, and she tried what was at the time this experimental technique. After seven days in the hospital, she had a stroke. I could tell that her condition had deteriorated significantly, and I took her home—against the advice of the neurologist and neurosurgeon. No more research, no more needles in her spine. Then, I placed her in hospice and the nurse came every day.

Even in those last months that Mami was so sick, she always used to tell me, "When I look at you, you give me so much confidence." This from a woman who in my eyes always favored my brother. But now she was telling me that I gave her confidence. That she thought anything can come her way and her daughter was going to get it done. That was a big compliment that my mother gave me. She had never been very affectionate and had lived by the words, "Be empathetic, not sympathetic." But here she was so confident that I could handle anything and everything. I cried when I left the room, and from that moment on did everything I could to make her life better. What a feeling of accomplishment I then had, but how sad that it had come so near the end.

Then she got a cold and by late afternoon she was going downhill. I had a board meeting at the University of Michigan that morning and I went. At noon, I got a call from the woman who cared for Mami saying that something was wrong with my mother, that she was calling my name constantly, constantly. "Please, can you come back?" the woman asked. I was now frantic, and there were not many planes from Detroit to Orlando. I got to the Detroit airport, and I was on standby. The woman behind the ticket counter looked at me, and I'm not sure if it was my face or my eyes or my body language, but she got me on a connecting flight to Orlando. Usually, I sit at the window seat over the wings, but on this flight, I was in the middle seat of the last row. I didn't care. I just wanted to get home. I landed, got to my car, and I drove home fast. Generally, when I speed, I get stopped by a police officer. No officer stopped me. I got home. The people from hospice were there. My friends were there. The woman who cleans the house was there. And there was my mother with her mouth open. I looked at her and I knew it was the end. Just like in the movies.

So I called Tomas and said, "Speak to her. She is in her last moments, and I want her to hear your voice." I left the room so that they could have privacy. I called her best friend, Ketty, from Puerto Rico—the one who would come and stay a week with her. She was the junior high school librarian, and she was able to say good-bye to my mother. The hospice man was there, and he was reading from the Bible and singing and humming in the most beautiful way. Anna, the lady who had helped take care of her, lay down on her left side and I was on the right side. We were almost like a sandwich, keeping her warm. I whispered in her ear that it was okay to go—that I was going to be okay, and she didn't need to worry about me. She could go in peace. I held one of her hands, Anna held the other one. She died at seven a.m. on October 9, 2010. She passed so quietly. And I cried.

I sent her to the funeral home that I had selected when she was going downhill. Anna and I gave her a bath and put her in a bright, beautiful set of pajamas. They came to pick her up and as they were leaving with her, I said, please cover her with a blanket, I don't want her to get cold. She was going to a refrigerator, and I was thinking that I didn't want her to get cold. Mami had chosen what she was to wear—and what should be in her casket. It had to be red. She asked me to put her favorite blanket at the end of her coffin. I put her favorite purse in there, too, as well as her favorite little toy animal and a coin purse containing a picture of every one of her grandchildren. I even put a little money in the coin purse. You never know!

Mami's body was flown to Puerto Rico; I was on the same flight. Even though she loved flowers, when we arrived in Fajardo it was a holiday, and no flowers could be found—everything was closed in my hometown. We ordered the flowers instead from the capital city of San Juan and they arrived—all of them red.

It was a wonderful ceremony. She was buried with very deserving honors. She had a beautiful mass before the burial. The Mayor spoke about her impressive life and the contributions she made. The Teacher's Association of Puerto Rico sang the teachers' song and draped her coffin with the Puerto Rican flag and the teachers' flag. I spoke. Tomas spoke as well. To this day, her grave has four dozen red roses that are changed monthly. Red is her color even in death.

Mami was a very sharp dresser. She had said, "When I die, make sure that your three nieces pick whatever they want. Give choices to my friend Ketty and to my friend Aida. Everything else, you are going to let my teachers come in here and pick exactly what they want, from my shoes to my purses to my clothes." And that is exactly how it happened. They went through her things and took what they wanted. The little that was left when they were done, I donated.

I have no regrets about the care that I gave Mami in those last months of her life. I worked as hard as I could during the hours I was at work at the hospital. When I was with her in the evenings and on weekends, it was just her in my life. Whatever she wanted. The bonding that occurred during that time made up for what had not happened in the years before. Even now, there are many days when I say I have to tell that to Mami, and then I remember that she is gone.

When she died, I cried briefly at that moment. Two weeks later, I cried uncontrollably and this time for one whole day. I don't know why. I guess it finally hit me. Now, I miss her tremendously and wish I could share with her the many things that have happened in my life since she has been gone. But I know somewhere along the way that she knows. So even after her death, I keep accomplishing things because she always had this trust that I would be somebody. And so a part of me doesn't want to disappoint her.

After Mami's death, Tomas and I became estranged. I thought that he had not given my mother the importance she deserved when she was in Orlando. There were many Sundays when I knew she was expecting either him or his daughters to come or call—and nothing happened. She would hold her pain and never utter a word, but I could see it in her eyes.

I had even told Mami, "When you are gone, I think our family will not be the same." And she said, "I know, and I understand where you are coming from. I myself have given up on some of them." I also told her I was leaving my estate to the University of Michigan so that women—specifically minorities—could study medicine. She said she understood that decision as well.

Despite the partial estrangement with Tomas, I have always helped him and his family members whenever they needed medical attention—referring them to the best that medicine can offer for their particular ailment. I feel that I am the surrogate mother to his three daughters. This is because the women on their maternal side have all died. Their mother died of cancer. Their grandmother died of cancer. Their aunt died of cancer. So I am really the only family they have besides their father. Through my nieces, I have three grandnephews.

My friend Cid Wilson alerted me in 2020 that I had been named one of the 100 Women of the Century by *USA Today*. I opened the article, thinking that it was all a joke, and there I was right in the middle of the women who had been recognized in the science category. Very close to my picture were those of the three NASA women from the book and movie *Hidden Figures*. I promised that I would do my best to honor the award and live up to the expectations of those who had selected me. I am grateful and still humbled by this award and its element of surprise, and I remember some famous words that I thought were appropriate at the time:

Talent is God-given. Be humble.
Fame is man-given. Be grateful.
Conceit is self-given. Be careful.

When Tomas learned of this honor, he called me with a message that was very poignant. I could feel that he was crying. I was so overjoyed that the sensitive Tomas was back. He even said, "I wish that Mami were here to feel as proud as I am of all your endeavors." Since then, I still do not visit his house, but I never forget to call him for birthdays, Father's Day, and Christmas. I hope time will take care of my feelings and disappointments regarding my family. Who knows, at the end, it could be back to normal.

* * *

Since my retirement, I have been able to provide much humanitarian and medical support to Puerto Rico. I have spent a minimum of two weeks each month there for the past six years.

Hurricane Irma and, two weeks later, Hurricane Maria inflicted tremendous damage on the Island of Puerto Rico during September of 2017. As I heard about the sadness and devastation, I wanted to get to the island to help. I couldn't. There were no flights between Florida and Puerto Rico, and the airport in San Juan was closed. Five Puerto Rican emergency doctors from Florida Hospital Orlando (now AdventHealth) were able to get to the island at the end of September. Through those connections, I arrived the first week of October along with about two thousand pounds of medical material, including sorely needed cardiovascular equipment.

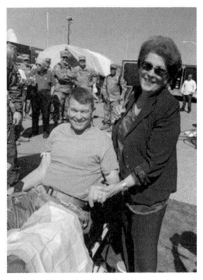

The Florida Hospital Orlando team welcomed me with open arms and took me with them to the Hyatt House San Juan where they were staying. At times, four of us women slept in the same room at the hotel, which became our home and the place where we felt comfortable after working so hard during the day, visiting and working in any hospital that needed help.

Dr. Novello and General Jeffrey Buchanan during an emergency drill after Hurricane Maria.

Immediately upon our arrival, the government of Puerto Rico issued each of us a temporary medical license number so that we could deliver services.

The preponderance of dead trees, dead animals, and fallen power lines made travel on any of the roads quite difficult. I threw my three-star weight around as a former Surgeon General and spoke with the Army General in charge of hurricane relief for Puerto Rico, General Jeffrey Buchanan, a three-star as well. He gave us his blessing to use military helicopters for medical relief. With that help, we visited close to fifty emergency rooms in as many towns and saved quite a few lives—especially people suffering from trauma and those needing insulin.

Once the USNS *Comfort* medical ship arrived in Puerto Rico, it became the place where everyone went for consultation, X-rays, and hospitalization. Many primary care doctors on the island were upset that their patients were attending the tent clinics of the USNS *Comfort* instead of coming to their offices. However, with no electricity, no internet, and no way to charge visits or call on the phone, this was the best way to provide medical services in the short term. And the patients took advantage of the opportunity.

Everywhere we went we found people begging for food and water. We carried food and water provided by FEMA and military rations from the National Guard and helped distribute them. That food also became our food when we were stranded in the field and unable to fly. The electrical storms were huge and frequent; the chief pilot would not risk disaster in any shape or form.

We did what we needed to do, and in the first months—with two of the humanitarian teams—we had visited close to fifty of the seventy-eight towns in Puerto Rico.

When the Advent teams left, I worked with a group of engineers from a company named PACIV. PACIV employees were altruistic, and they had received donations of $1 million from pharmaceutical companies for the relief effort that needed to be efficiently distributed. We evaluated the needs of the very sick and poor in need of emergency ambulance transfer to the States. We sent many people to the continental US for multiple issues—cancer therapies, tumors, head traumas, infections, and the like. Each ambulance ride cost $29,000, and a family member, the pilot, and the patient were the ones in the cabin. If someone was extremely ill, a nurse would also be part of the transfer team. Upon arrival, Florida Senator Marco Rubio's office in Orlando, through his Director Elena Crosby, served as the liaison to get them to their next step in medical treatment and, for some, getting them into the Medicaid system. All of us together saved quite a few people this way.

We were also in charge of buying and installing huge electric generators in neighborhoods so people would have some form of electricity. Donations helped extend the original budget, and we helped many people—some with extreme burns—transfer to the Puerto Rico Medical Center, San Juan City Hospital, for care.

The first patient we saved was very special to us. A little boy with enzymatic deficiency—Diego—whose medication was not available in Puerto Rico. We found just one dose, bought it, administered it, and immediately sent him to Orlando for care in the air ambulance. Today he is alive and thriving, and we communicate with his mother frequently.

As the major crises of the storm became more manageable, I decided to share my expertise with another group, VOCES, which was in charge of vaccinating against influenza. It was at this time that the group of PACIV of which I was a part also started helping a doctor in the western part of the island seeing patients in the priest's office, next to a church. He had little medication for his many patients. Through the US Army, Senator Rubio's office, and Elena Crosby, we were able to provide him with a portable military tent hospital—with air conditioning and a supply of medications. This became a local hospital in the town of Aguada for a long time, until the emergency was over.

We also helped establish a clinic in the town of Utuado, serving eight barrios. It took between two and three hours to get there every day to take medications, cots, blankets, and food for them. We were able to accommodate their needs with the help of volunteers (Fermin Arraiza in particular), good faith, and the National Guard medical team. In Utuado, Tito Valentin, the owner of the local gas station, had requested help. He had supplies of every kind in his gas station including Women, Infants, and Children's (commonly known as WIC) supplies. He and his volunteer COSSAO crew helped construct the clinic, the roads, and the bridges, and eventually he knew the name of each person who lived in the barrios. Universities started sending teams to be trained there, and the Puerto Rico National Guard canceled their Christmas vacation to start treating patients there in a tent and a one-room clinic. When the clinic was expanded to two rooms, we gave the number of the National Guard units as their room name—the Guard loved the honor. The clinic eventually grew to accommodate every service that any hospital in the capital city could offer but with a sense of pride and ownership. It now has an ambulance, an emergency room, a large dental clinic, and a mental health clinic. In addition, gynecological services are provided, including pap smears and breast cancer screening. It even has a medical director! For his outstanding humanitarian efforts, leadership, and community involvement, Tito Valentin won the Honoris Causa award from the University Central del Caribe Medical School.

In the beginning of my humanitarian work in Puerto Rico, my lodging was paid for by VOCES during the influenza vaccination campaign. It is now being paid for by the Society for Education and Rehabilitation (SER). This organization services children and adults with disabilities. I was able to get them a certification to become a vaccination clinic for their clients. Every child they serve has now been vaccinated, which I find very satisfying and fulfilling.

After the duty for all of us was somewhat finalized, I was able to devise an award for about fifty people and/or groups involved in the humanitarian mission. It was called the US Surgeon General Award—Angels of Maria. I loved the feeling and camaraderie that came about, despite all the destruction. At the same time, I requested and obtained permission to give a humanitarian ribbon for service during Maria to all those public health officers assigned to Puerto Rico during the emergency. The ribbons were awarded during a wonderful ceremony at the HHS building.

After the January 2020 earthquake in Puerto Rico, I received a call from General José Reyes, the General in charge of the Puerto

Rico National Guard. He was calling to inquire if I wanted to assist in the aftermath of the earthquake. People in five towns were sleeping in front of their homes—afraid of aftershocks or another earthquake and wanting to protect their properties.

Of course, I said yes. Every day we went by helicopter to visit five tent cities. We checked to verify that they had enough food and that no one was sick. We inspected the latrines and went to the tent where the sickest people were being treated. At one point, rain flooded two of the tent camps and they had to be rebuilt.

It was quite an experience. Puerto Rico had not in recent memory had an earthquake. Many people still fear the aftershocks. To this moment, they continue to happen across the south of the island, but in smaller magnitudes.

Two hurricanes, an earthquake, and then a pandemic. The National Guard, as always, was prepared. Once the vaccine became available during the pandemic, VOCES and the National Guard worked to vaccinate the people of Puerto Rico. Puerto Rico became number one in the US in the percentage of the population that had been vaccinated because of these combined efforts.

I have received two awards recognizing my service—the medal from the National Guard for Humanitarian work during Maria and the Sister Isolina Ferré Medal for service to the community. The biggest recognition, however, came from the average Puerto Rican in the streets after a group of anti-vaxxers wanted to smear my reputation on the news by bringing up my issue in New York. I was beyond anger, but I did not stay quiet. I spoke my piece! Anti-vaxxers were outside of the studio screaming profanities, and some of us needed protection to leave the building. The morning after, I went to a street in the center of the capital city to return something. It was unreal. The cars beeping as they passed me by. The people on the sidewalks touching or hugging me, saying "Doctora, don't worry about those crazy ones," and the most touching of all—three young men in a bar door screaming, "Doctora, we love you!"

Just when I thought I was not valued because of someone's negative comments, people came alive to support me. They served as my cocoon of affection to protect me so that I would not be harmed. This experience taught me that love and respect from your people is more important than a paper diploma or a silver medal!

In early 2020, I was on my way to Puerto Rico. On the flight, the attendant asked if there was a doctor in the house. I thought to myself, *No way, Jose, I have answered this call enough times.* I saw a doctor pass by and said, "Thank you, God." But the commotion kept getting bigger. I was in the window seat, and I asked the woman in the aisle seat what seemed to be the problem. She said, "I don't know, but there is a child on the floor." I immediately got up and tried to help. The flight attendant said, "I'm sorry we are busy, you cannot go through here." I said that I was a pediatrician, she let me pass, and I saw the other doctor giving oxygen to the baby. I knelt beside the other doctor and said, "You do what you have to do. I will ask the parents some questions." He agreed. I asked the parents if the child had been vaccinated recently. I asked if the child had been screaming when she was eating. I asked about medications and if the child had a cold. I told the doctor I thought she had had an aspiration (when fluid or liquids enter the airway or the lungs by accident) because when the mother changed the baby's diaper, she had also given her milk, and the baby cried at the same time.

We told the pilot that, when we landed, we would need an ambulance for the baby to be taken to the hospital. When I was going back to my seat, the doctor turned around and gave me his name and said, "Thank you for taking care of this." He asked my name, and I said Dr. Novello. He went into shock—"WHAT? You're Dr. Novello?" He said thank you for saving my life because I am a urologist. When we were leaving the plane, he wanted a picture of the two of us. Beautiful memories. The baby did have aspiration pneumonia and did well.

In 2021, I was asked to be the Secretary of Health of Puerto Rico by the currently constitutionally appointed Governor of Puerto Rico. However, some concerns were raised that my conviction in New York made me ineligible. I was told the Governor would consult with her legal team. After I was interviewed for the position and was waiting for a decision, I saw on television that a new Secretary of Health had been named—it was not me. No one had contacted my attorney or me. I believe that God decided that my skills could be better used elsewhere. Time has proven that was not the job for me. God is great!

* * *

Thirteen years after my New York conviction, March 31, 2022, I got news that my legal case had been sealed—closed, finished. Free at last. Thank God, I am free at last. I felt vindicated from what many top-ranking government officials considered the biggest case of entrapment that they had ever witnessed.

This part of my life has taught me many lessons—which I excerpt from *Leadership Secrets of Attila the Hun* by Dr. Wess Roberts:

"Be wise and anticipate the Brutus of your camp.
You will always be double crossed by those closest to you.
The envy from your peers will increase as you excel."

But I believe in my heart of hearts that karma never forgets your address.

* * *

Sometimes when you love, you do things that other people think are crazy, or they criticize you for those behaviors.

Joe and I were divorced in 1994, but we lived together in the Georgetown house until 1998 when it sold, everything was finalized, and we finally went our separate ways. We spoke regularly on the phone after that, often when he was driving to or from work. In

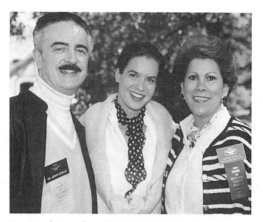

*Dr. Joseph Novello and Dr. Antonia Novello at the
Academy of Achievement with Olympic champion
figure skater Katarina Witt.*

1998, when I won the Hispanic Heritage Awards—Leadership Award
from the Kennedy Center, he hosted a brunch for me and my friends,
wrote my speech, and there he was in the second row with all of Puerto
Rico. When I did the commencement speech for Hopkins and got my
doctorate in public health (2000), he sent me two dozen white roses.
When I was accused by the Albany 5, Joe was on the phone asking me
to go to their country home to be away from everything.

In April of 2021, it didn't surprise me that he called me and
asked for help, and I gave it. He was not feeling well. I assumed
it could have been a mild stroke or long-term COVID since he
had tested positive for COVID maybe two months before. I took
him and his wife to the Mayo Clinic in Jacksonville, Florida, and
a tumor on the right side of his brain, called a gliosarcoma, stage
IV, was diagnosed. The tumor was successfully removed, and he
received chemotherapy and radiation at the University of Virginia
hospital in Charlottesville, Virginia. In early 2022, he had been free
of the tumor for months and he moved to an assisted living facility
in McLean, Virginia. I visited and tended to him at that facility,

seven to ten days each month—together with friends and other members of his family.

My behavior has been criticized by some. I don't care. If you love someone and he needs your help—you help. Especially when that person asks for help, and Joe asked for mine. I would not abandon him to his fate—I would not let him die in indignity. I promised him that. Whenever there were moments of doubt regarding my presence at this time in his life, I just looked at him and remembered the good times, his patting my head every time I did something for him, his "I love you" every time he went into a surgical procedure, and the look in his eyes when we were alone in his room talking. I would never leave him or disappoint him. I could not live with the pain or guilt.

All through Joe's illness, I did not allow myself to feel—afraid of the looks among strangers—especially since he was married, and if he recovered, he would pick up his life where he had left it before his diagnosis. I was not going to suffer from Joe's abandonment twice in my life. I stayed until the end and never showed my pain. To this day, I have not shed a tear.

I am so tired of watching the people I love die. First my mother, then Joe's parents, and now Joe. I was somewhat ready for Mami and the Novellos to die, but even though I knew it had to come, Joe's death caught me by surprise. His body, communication skills, and his ability to walk or even use his walker all came to a halt sometime between February and March 2023. His mind was very clear, and even though his spoken words were very hard to understand at times, he was communicating with hands, hugs, blown kisses, and smiles. Then his confusion grew intermittently, and his favorite priest came, held mass, and gave him his final blessing—communion and last rites. Upon the priest's departure, Joe grabbed his hand and kissed it. We all became teary. What a gesture from a dying man—so dignified and thoughtful until the end.

His coughing accompanied by shortness of breath, with oxygen prongs needed, became more pronounced and almost constant. Then came the hardest part of his dying—his wailing, painfully constant, loud, and with moments of agony in his face and demeanor. I asked him if he was in pain—he moved his head and meant no, but when I asked him why the wailing, out of his mouth that had not spoken coherently for almost three to four days came, "I don't know!" It just crumbled me. I, who was supposed to know how to help people, couldn't help him! They gave him a medication for anxiety and some morphine, and when it seemed he could rest, someone would come in the room wanting to connect with him, which sadly meant more morphine more frequently.

At the end was what I call the "litany of I'm sorrys," I'm sorry I should have called. I'm sorry I didn't come. Each interruption that Joe endured near the end woke him up and caused him to experience pain and require another shot of morphine. In the following twenty-four hours, he had gotten so much morphine that his respirations were diminishing in time and length. I had stayed with him all night, holding his hand and placing my other one inside his pajamas so that I could detect his breathing problems and the awaited final breath by touching his chest and his ribs.

Around 4:45 a.m., I knew something was about to happen—his demeanor was exactly like Mami's before she died, and I left the room, went to my room to get my blood pressure medicine—because I knew I was going to need some help. When I came back, he had just died, at 5:38 a.m. I could not even think of why I went to look for my pills when I missed his parting by less than fifty minutes! I am consoled thinking that he died when I wasn't there so that I didn't have to watch it happen. This was a hard moment in my life—the loneliness of my soul, the pain in my heart, and no one to cry with (except Kojo—his male nurse companion of months) who understood how I felt. I have never felt so alone in my life! Joe was no longer there to protect me from strangers—and suddenly his family came and took over everything without acknowledging my presence. No one ever thanked me for taking care of him—even when that was not my responsibility. I know he would have protected me, but in his absence, I did not shed a tear. I just took over myself and finished the last job: placing him, with the help of the funeral personnel, in a black bag with a zipper, and that's when my heart closed to pain and tears. I left the room after the hearse left.

Joe's death taught me many things. First, do all you need and want to do while the person you love is alive! Don't show your love by tears and screaming—that person won't be able to hear you—but give them hugs, kisses, and company when they need them the most.

Don't lie or make promises you will not keep. We must respect our loved ones even when they are unaware of some of the promises we made.

Answer questions with the truth—but make it understandable and kind. Never be final in the assessments, and always give hope. Who are we to play God?

Help your loved one pray, even in a state of semiconsciousness—that person needs to come close with their spirituality, and their God.

Find a priest or a layperson that occasionally stops by their bedside and reminds them to acknowledge their own mortality, but at the same time helps them have peace with their parting. It's inevitable, death, but it surely helps make the journey faster, more peaceful, and acceptable to both them and us.

> **"Do all you need and want to do while the person you love is alive!"**

I have no regrets about all the things I had to endure as the ex-wife during these almost last two years of Joe's life. I didn't push myself on him. He was the one who contacted me. And since that day, my biggest and happiest moments were those when he would tell me, just like my mother, that I gave him confidence, and that I got things done for him and—only in our private moments—that he loved me, especially before any surgical procedures. And I would tell him in return: "I will always be here, I will not abandon you or not care for you—you will not suffer indignities while I'm with you, and you will die in peace when the day comes." And so it was.

When you love, you love.

* * *

With a life as rich and full as mine, there are many stories, lessons learned, regrets, and other thoughts. So many people have asked me which job I liked best—US Surgeon General or Commissioner of the Department of Health of the State of New York. That is not an easy question to answer. The Surgeon General is the spokesperson for the nation, recommended by a society group or important person to the President, confirmed by the US Senate for a four-year term, and serving under the Office of Secretary of HHS. The only one who can fire the Surgeon General is the President.

The job of Commissioner of Health is different in so many ways. That position is recommended by the Governor of the State of New York and confirmed by the New York Senate. The length of term is dependent on the number of years that Governor, or the subsequent Governor, is in office. In addition, the New York Commissioner of Health has the power and the money to back up their agenda. One-third of the budget of the state of New York falls under the Department of Health. In addition, many important subdivisions are under the umbrella of the department.

In reality, I enjoyed my job as Commissioner more than my job as US Surgeon General. There was so much more variety, from hospitals and nursing home supervision to approving certificates of need to supervision of laboratories, blood banks, and funeral parlors. A few of the additional responsibilities included drafting policies for new diseases and keeping track of doctors' licenses and behaviors.

However, as I also say, once a Surgeon General, always a Surgeon General. In the course of history, there have only been twenty-one Surgeons General in one hundred years, all men except for three women.

It seems that many of the important events that have happened in my life and that changed my future I either read about in the newspaper, heard on the radio, or saw on television. I was driving toward Constitution Avenue in Washington, D.C., when I heard on the radio that I had been confirmed by the US Senate to be Surgeon General. No calls from the government, the White House, nothing. Similarly, I heard on the radio and then saw on television that Dr. Joycelyn Elders was going to replace me as Surgeon General. It was not until about two weeks later that I heard from the incoming Secretary of HHS in a personal phone call. And I learned about the charges against me in New York State by reading about them in the *New York Times*. It all seems very odd to me.

I remember three specific times in my life where my Vice Admiral rank made a difference.

The first was early in my Surgeon General tenure. I was getting my uniform with my new rank at the Navy shop in Bethesda, and a seamstress was helping me by sewing my stripes on my jacket. While she was stitching very slowly an officer was behind me waiting and shuffling her feet constantly as if she were in a rush. I believe this other officer thought she was being held up by me, an officer junior to her, and that I was a mere two stripe (LT JG—Lieutenant Junior Grade) while she had three stripes. As she was about to push in front of me the seamstress started stitching—not the two small stripes but the big one. So together there were three stripes, but not of a Lieutenant but of a Vice Admiral! The officer left in a rush, and I had my uniform finished and ready to wear for the first time the next morning.

The second time, I went to the VA Hospital to look for my medical records. In every VA Hospital there is always an enlisted man or retired veteran directing the public where they want to go. I indicated that I was looking for medical records, and the man pointed to a closed door. I waited for a while by the door, but when no one came out or went in, I asked another person where the medical records would be found. This man said that they were located in the back in trailers, and he proceeded to accompany me there.

When we got to the trailers, there were two young guys sitting in chairs with their feet propped on the front desk. I had given the person who was helping me my ID card as we walked. When we arrived in front of the desk, he looked at my ID card, and with a puzzled look on his face he asked me, "What is RA RA?" To which I said, "RA RA? I don't know what you mean." He showed my ID to me, and I said, "Oh, that is Rear Admiral." To which he immediately stood at attention and said, "Attention on Deck." The two guys moved so swiftly that they almost fell out of their chairs to stand up and stand at attention. They not only found my record instantly they also proceeded to accompany me to my car. I loved my rank that day!

The third occasion was when the USNS *Comfort* came to Puerto Rico to help during the aftermath of Hurricane Maria. The USNS *Comfort* was a huge war ship sent to take care of medical emergencies. Since there was hardly any electricity functioning on the island, most medical offices weren't able to bring up patient medical records, use their computers, or do a billing. Most Puerto Ricans used the USNS *Comfort* as a medical clinic. I wanted to see it, but the Secretary of Health of Puerto Rico never had the time to take me. So I decided to take myself.

I went to where the ship was anchored, and I saw a very large enlisted man in front of a podium, guarding the entrance. I approached him and said, "Sir, I would like to come aboard to see the USNS *Comfort* and its capabilities." He looked at me like I was an alien and asked in a very patronizing way, "Ma'am how many lines do you have on your jacket?" (I am a petite woman, and I was wearing jeans and a blouse.) And I said, "Lines? What do you mean?" And, he said, "You heard me, lines." And I said, "You mean like rank?" And he nodded. And I said I have one big one and two little ones. I didn't even have my ID with me, but he stood at attention and said, "Attention on Deck! Call the Captain."

Needless to say, I saw the USNS *Comfort* inch by inch, and then I was escorted out. And I thanked the man who almost blocked my entrance. Always a lady and an officer!

Mami dressed well and taught me to do the same. I believe that you should dress the best that you can, especially for an interview, because your curriculum vitae will not be enough. The first impression is critically important, and there is no do-over.

I will always remember a researcher with a terrific curriculum vitae who came to interview when I was at the NIH. She arrived at the interview wearing a bomber jacket, jeans, and a Stetson hat with a huge feather. I knew her attire would seriously impact how she was perceived, so I very diplomatically asked her to leave her hat in my office and if she would be willing to wear the black jacket that was always on the hanger on the back of my office door. She took off the hat and wore my jacket for the interview and got the job of her life. She still works at NIH.

Here are a few other remembrances that I would like to share.

Governor Pataki approached me while I was Commissioner to run against Hillary Clinton for Senator. The Republicans needed a throwaway candidate. I told him that I didn't want to be the canary in the cage and that I didn't have the money or the interest in pursuing the position. He understood and found someone else. The rest is history.

One of Joe's very close friends became the attaché to the embassy in Rome. We were fortunate to visit with him when he was stationed in Rome, and he was able to get us into the Sistine Chapel at the Vatican when it was undergoing renovation. I felt like Michelangelo with scaffolding everywhere. On top of the scaffolding was the high extended hand of God—no cameras were allowed but what an amazing feeling as I touched it!

One of my most embarrassing life experiences had to do with the aftereffects of my congenital megacolon surgery at age eighteen. Some of these effects, albeit rare, I continue to experience to this day. Over time, I have become very intolerant to a variety of foods, including onions, cream, cabbage, and some oils. There was one resulting incident that took me completely by surprise. Joe and I were at a black-tie dinner at the national association of pilots who are physicians convention in Chicago. The President of the association was giving his speech and at the end, everybody stood up for a standing ovation. And suddenly, I said to myself, this cannot be happening to me. I looked at my husband and I said, "Joe, Joe." He said, "What?" Then he looked down at me and saw that I was covered in brown liquid all the way to my ankles. I never felt anything—it must have been something I ate.

I said, "Joe, what am I going to do?" He said that we should wait until the people go up to the President and start celebrating, and then when we were alone, I could go to the bathroom. When I got to the bathroom, there were many other women waiting in line, so I took an elevator to the second floor. Everyone was looking at me, and I said that a little girl puked on me.

I got to the stall and cleaned myself up the best that I could. The inner parts of my gown were really messed up, so I took the lining off and washed it. Women would walk in while I was doing all of this, and I could see from their faces that there was quite a smell. I put my gown back on and I said, "Joe, we're leaving." Everyone, including us, had come on a bus, but Joe and I were walking on the sidewalk. All the people on the bus were yelling, "Toni and Joe, come on and get on the bus." We said, "No, we're going to walk." The bus left and Joe hailed a taxi. We were so thankful to be in a cab, but the cab driver—not so much. He lowered all the windows because of the smell. I was so embarrassed.

When we returned to our room, I dropped into the tub with my clothes on. I washed them and then put on another formal gown—to attend a reception at our hotel. When we walked into the reception, people commented how sassy I was—two formal gowns in the same night. Back in our room that night we laughed so hard. Joe didn't laugh easily but he did, thinking that the mess left behind might be considered chocolate mousse!

At future gatherings, when I wanted to leave a situation, I would look at Joe and I would say, "Joe, I think Chicago is coming." He knew exactly what it meant, and he would grudgingly leave with me. But once he caught on that it wasn't real, I couldn't use the excuse any longer.

I was boarding the plane to fly back to the US from the Dominican Republic during the time I was serving as a consultant to the US Embassy on issues of domestic violence. I noticed that unusual attention was being directed toward my passport. I asked if anything was the matter and they said not to worry, it would be handled at customs. At the departure area, two police—one woman and one man—stopped me and asked me to go with them. Naturally, I was concerned, but you do not show any disrespect for law, especially in a foreign country. In addition, one of them had a dog, and I became concerned that they suspected me of transporting drugs.

After about twenty minutes, the policewoman approached me, and I asked her if I should contact the US Embassy. She went back to talk to customs and the other police officer before coming back to tell me that they thought I had a false passport. I said I had better call the embassy. She said, Doña (Madam), we believe that this passport is false because you look much too good to be the age that it says you are.

I didn't know if I wanted to laugh, accept the compliment, or slap her. Now that I understood the issue, however, I showed her other pictures, including my government ID that showed my picture with my name. She accepted all the documents that I showed her.

She congratulated me again for looking so good for my age and let me board the plane. What a relief.

It's a nice thing to be able to flaunt the Legion of Merit. When you are in the military, your curriculum vitae is on your chest. Many years ago, when I was Surgeon General, there was a question in one of the newspapers or *Parade* magazine: Does the Surgeon General have all those ribbons to match her lipstick? Would anyone ask such a question if the Surgeon General were a man? Really, am I less than a man because I am a woman that has medals? Right now, I was told that I am the Public Health Service officer with the most ribbons. Why? Because I am the only US Surgeon General who is alive who was a true career Public Health Officer. Many Surgeons General were from universities, and when their term as Surgeon General was over, they returned to academia. I returned to the NIH and then to UNICEF. I have twenty-six years of service medals on my uniform. I have ten rows each containing three ribbons. I am not chopped liver!

Now, when I go to meetings with the other Surgeons General, they say things to me like, "Honey, you are loaded." I say, "Honey, I am career." We like to kid each other a lot. And they respect me because I followed Dr. Koop. I get a little bit of respect for such a proud connection.

For more than fourteen years, I have survived the felony conviction in New York. I have continued to get invitations to speak. People still trust me. I have used the years since the conviction to rise above that. It is not going to distract me from doing what is right for the people.

I went to give a commencement speech in Massachusetts ten years after the New York conviction. The host picked me up at the airport and said, "I don't want you to be upset, but there is a press release about your felony in New York, and the President of the college is having doubts about you giving the commencement speech." I said to myself, *I am not going to let these people get me down—ten years after.* This reminded me of when I filled out the application to join the Public Health Service, and they didn't want to hire me because I had had therapy for marital issues. I went straight to the President and said, "You want to judge me? Put me in front of a group." I spoke to high schoolers. Then I went and spoke to the junior high and elementary students. I gave the commencement speech and got a standing ovation. Don't judge people by what you read, judge people by what they do.

As I look back now, I know I could have avoided so many problems in life if I had had a mentor to guide me. In college, I didn't know to take some of the "easier" courses since the credit counts were the same and I might have been able to increase my grade average. I was taking hard scientific courses because I thought that would be better preparation for medicine. Can you image the genetics of the tsetse fly instead of music appreciation? Go figure. And I didn't feel capable enough, so I also needed to enhance my own perception and standing. In addition, I didn't know when I walked into my medical school entrance test that everyone else had the Kaplan study guide. I didn't know that you could study for this kind of test. I don't even know how God helped me pass the MCAT, but I did. I was also intimidated by all the premed students because everyone was a top-notch science major or their father and/or mother was in the medical field.

I learned if you always complain about something and you don't do what you think you need to do, then you are the problem, not the solution itself. I learned to bypass the ones who are giving you problems or lateralize. I step aside so that you're not hitting me with your anger or with your hate.

I have lateralized at two major breakpoints in my life. I lateralized to keep away from the scorn, from the ones who criticized me, from the ones who said, "You cannot do it." You move out of their way—not to die, but to keep building away from the eyes of those who want to keep you down. I lateralized to get to a better place and to avoid challenges that I didn't think I could take on at the time. After you have learned what you need to learn, you can come back and tell those you have bypassed, "Do you remember me, I used to be in the back?" Usually, they have already forgotten you—out of sight, out of mind. I have built a stronger foundation and gained knowledge that I needed to move forward.

I know it is time to lateralize when I want to cry. I only cry at sad movies. I don't cry out of pain; I cry because I want to beat you up. Remember, there will be a light at the end of the tunnel if you endeavor to find it. But you cannot find it instantly; you have to work for it. Do not use time as a constraint. Time will pass, regardless of whether you act.

I lateralized when I was in grant management at the NIH. I had a female boss who complained that I had taken one of her Perrier waters out of the refrigerator. This was ridiculous as the secretary had given me the water, and the secretary was the one who bought the water and stocked the refrigerator. I looked for another job immediately. When I found that job, which was all PhDs and no MDs except for me, she told me that I was going there "to expire or retire." In the five years that I was in that job, I learned a tremendous amount regarding bone and kidney research in the United States and built a very strong network and knowledge base. Because of the experience I gained, I was ready to be Deputy of the National Institute for Child Health for

> "Remember, there will be a light at the end of the tunnel if you endeavor to find it."

the NIH. That probably wouldn't have happened if I hadn't lateralized. Later, I asked that former boss to cowrite a paper with me. However, she didn't meet the deadlines. I wrote the paper without her.

I came up at an earlier time when there were very few women in leadership positions. Unfortunately, many of those women were competitive and sabotaged each other instead of working collaboratively and helping other women climb the ladder. I call it opening the window

"Preparation meets opportunity equals success."

for others. I hope that workplace conditions are much better today. It was at moments like those that Mother's words came back in my ears: always study with men. They will not consider you to be competition—they will help you instead.

One of the reasons I studied public health was because I wanted to do good for the world even though no one knew that I existed in making the world better. Preparation meets opportunity equals success. I think young people need to understand that even if they have an elite education, what is important is what you are going to do with that education for yourself, your country, and your community.

Many years after my first surgery at the Mayo Clinic, I gave the commencement speech at the Mayo Clinic Medical School. People knew that I would always feel grateful to the Mayo. I still say regularly, but for the Mayo Clinic, I would not be where I am today. I called the male doctors at the Mayo "Brooks Brothers"—they always wore suits and ties, not the white coats. As I was giving my commence-

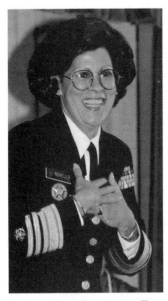

Portrait of a smiling Dr. Novello.

ment speech, a little boy, maybe two and a half years old, came running through the audience of students screaming, "Daddy, Daddy, Daddy." And I stopped the commencement. I looked at the graduating class and said, "Whose child is this?" The father sheepishly stood up. I said "Well, come over and pick up your kid, and let's make sure he is okay. Then we'll continue this graduation." So people started applauding, and he was in awe that we had interrupted the gradua-tion ceremony so that he could pick up his little baby he didn't even know was coming down the aisle. It's good to be a pediatrician because only then can you do something like that in the middle of the Mayo Clinic Medical School graduation.

More than half a century after my first surgery at the Mayo Clinic and considering all my life changes since then (travel, different foods, different countries, different schedules), I consider myself in good health mentally and physically. This is despite the occasional accident or the very infrequent utilization of an enema when the need arises. I feel blessed that none of this has interfered with my life routines. The Mayo Clinic is and always will be my place to go when I am in need. The appointments are kept on time, my records are never lost, and my diagnosis is shared with me during my stay. All in all, the Mayo Clinic rates a "10."

An organization that is also very important to me is the United States Hispanic Leadership Institute (USHLI). I have attended its meetings

> "Do good things and you will be remembered for your deeds."

for many years and have won two important awards from them—the National Hispanic Hero Award and the Dolores Huerta Woman of Courage Medallion.

In 2022, perhaps for my humanitarian work in Puerto Rico, USHLI established the Dr. Antonia C. Novello Humanitarian Medallion. What a privilege it was for me to bestow the medallion on the first two honorees in 2023. The evening at which I presented the award contained a surprise as well. Dr. Juan Andrade, Jr., the director of USHLI went to the podium to make his remarks. He was delighted to see everyone in person, and he reminded the audience that he had almost died of liver failure and that the person who had fought for his life and found a liver transplant for him was sitting in the audience—Dr. Antonia C. Novello. I had no words. Do good things and you will be remembered for your deeds—not for money or for accolades but for the joy of saving a life.

Epilogue

In this life of mine, I have had major disappointments, not to mention medical complications.

In spite of it all, I have had many successes, accolades, awards, and recognition as well. I am and have been grateful for all of these and for God's blessings, too.

Today, as I find myself in my seventies, I have come to realize that I have mostly lived to please society and others and in the process have forgotten about myself.

My jobs were important, and in some I excelled. In others I survived. But during the thirty years since I served as Surgeon General my life has been incomplete. Full of triumphs and responsibilities but devoid (except for a few) of human contact.

In my mind, I could not give myself that opportunity. My jobs were in the public eye, and I was not about to become the center of attention. I was to be centered only in service to others and public policy dealings.

In the twenty-eight years I have been divorced, I really never enjoyed a close relationship—under the mantra "I am not your nurse or your purse."

To this day, I still wear a wedding band. It keeps away the ones I am not interested in. I don't date. I don't even look to my right or left when my car is at the traffic light—I'm not interested in the view or the socialization.

And yet, I have laughed. I have also cried through some major disappointments. I have encountered new friends and wonderful colleagues, but I was always protecting the only thing that is mine: my persona and my privacy.

Writing this book has been a catharsis—transparency at all costs—privacy gone! I have told the truth while I have remembered and written about the past.

"I only wish I had spent more time loving, less time judging. More hugging, rather than distancing, which I did to protect myself from pain."

My hope in doing so is that through my life story, one day, there will be one woman, or one man, who will learn from my mistakes and survive the life surprises and friend abandonments without blaming only themselves.

I want them to use whatever is in this book to move ahead and be themselves.

My life has not been easy. But God, I would not change a thing.

I only wish I had spent more time loving, less time judging. More hugging, rather than distancing, which I did to protect myself from pain.

If there is another life to live, I will live it and participate more fully in what it has to offer—without fear. At seventy-nine years old, I am still here and living fully. I have not finished some of my life goals. I am working on them still. The best is yet to come.

Life Lessons and Rules to Live By

When you've lived a life as full as I have—with so many twists and turns—you accumulate some knowledge along the way and some advice to give others. Here is my top ten list. These ten points are accompanied by famous quotes from others and some excerpts from the book—*Dream Big! A Road Map for Facing Life's Challenges and Creating the Life You Deserve* by my friend Deborah Rosado Shaw.

NUMBER 10   Be a pioneer. Don't be afraid to forge into new directions.

When you think of pioneers, remember Rosa Parks, the seamstress who became the founding symbol of the civil rights movement in the US in 1955.

Her simple act of defiance in refusing to give up her seat on a bus changed our country. After her death, the Reverend Jesse Jackson, speaking on behalf of all African Americans, said it best: "She sat down in order that we might stand up."

So when you forge in new directions, remember, the ark was built by amateurs, the *Titanic* by professionals.

NUMBER 9   Do not deny your roots as you walk up the ladder of success.

For if you deny your roots, you have no integrity—you gave up your dignity.

Colleagues, nothing is worth the cost of your integrity, your reputation, or your self-respect.

If you cannot honor your racial, cultural, moral, and social concepts inherited from your ancestors, then how can you demand it from the rest?

Remember, people without knowledge of their origin or culture are like a tree without roots: they will fall over.

NUMBER 8   Never underestimate your capabilities; others will do it for you.

Remember—your most worthy efforts will be scorned by your peers, for it is they who suffer most when you excel.

Remember as well that as a chief achieves greater success, the jealousy others feel for him will intensify.

So do not squander your energy fighting every little skirmish—you will be depleted when you need to fight the important ones.

Ask yourself: Do I have enemies? Good—that means that you've stood up for something sometime in your life.

Additionally, as Eleanor Roosevelt said, remember that great people discuss ideas, average people discuss events, and little people discuss people. Remember this, too—a lion doesn't lose sleep over the opinions of sheep.

NUMBER 7   Achieve the highest level of education—it is the key to the door of opportunity.

While getting an education, remember, the complete professional must be humble in what facts they do not know!

Remember that Socrates said that if he was the most intelligent man in Greece, it's because he knew what he didn't know.

No matter how educated you are: never make a decision when you do not understand the issue. And above all, learn to say, "I don't know."

Remember as well, you do not have to be brilliant to be successful. As Michelango said. The greatest danger for most of us is not that our aim is too high, and we miss it, but that it is too low, and we reach it.

NUMBER
6
Set goals for yourself, and when doing so, make them realistic and then share them with those who believe in you.

In pursuing your goals, whenever you run into a wall, find a way of walking around it if you haven't learned how to knock it down.

Lament, if necessary, but do not dwell too long on your bad moments lest they rise to rule your emotions forever.

When you are unhappy at your work, do something about it—otherwise you become the problem, not the solution.

Remember, too, what Eleanor Roosevelt said: "No one can make you feel inferior without your consent." And as Rikkie Gale once said, "I used to walk into a room and wonder if they like me, now I look around in a room and wonder if I like them."

NUMBER
5
When you get to the top, don't forget you owe something back to your peers, your family, and your community.

And as a woman, when you get to the top, do not deliver the sermon of equality—live by it! By that I mean do not practice abuses of power, such as withholding information, leapfrogging through hierarchy, displacing deserving professionals, making unfulfilled promises, and not correcting salary inequities.

None of these should be used to keep a woman down—especially when the boss is you, a woman like me!

Equally as important: do not forget that being a leader is often a lonely job. So, if you want to be one, prepare for it!

But above all, remember "that most successes result from group efforts—so do not forget to network; you cannot do without it. It is a great way to increase your visibility and give your insight on the attitudes necessary to break into a new field."

NUMBER **4** **Don't be afraid to speak your mind. Remember to *first* be who you are and say what you feel because those who mind don't matter, and those who matter don't mind.**

Remember, too: be more concerned with your character than your reputation, because your character is what you really are while your reputation is merely what others think you are.

But as my friend Deborah says, "Don't get sucked into being the hero in your own life—whatever you do, do not use someone else's vision as a guide for your own life."

Above all:

- *Don't take everything personally.*
- *Be factual—not just emotional.*
- *Do not repeat the mistakes of your predecessors.*
- *Do not let disappointment drag you down.*
- *Be assertive without being bullish.*

NUMBER **3** **Take care of yourself spiritually, physically, and mentally. Remember, "we either make ourselves miserable or we make ourselves strong. After all, the amount of work is the same."**

Remember as well, when it comes to your own life, you don't have to get it right all the time. "Perfection is not required!"

"There is no reason to perpetuate the fantasy that we can fix it all, be it all, do it all, twenty-four hours a day, seven days a week!"

"So, take time to renew yourself and take a break:"

- *Read mindless novels.*
- *Take power naps.*
- *Have an ice cream without guilt.*
- *Get a manicure, a facial, lift weights.*
- *Turn your cell phone off and daydream!*

And above all, practice assertiveness:

- *Don't swallow the words you want—or need—to say.*
- *Get accustomed to sticking up for yourself as if you were your only best friend.*

NUMBER **2** **Never lose your sense of who you really are, even when others believe they know you better than you know yourself.**

As Judy Garland said, always be a first-rate version of yourself instead of a second-rate version of somebody else. You were born an original, so don't die a copy.

But, above all, never settle for just looking good—because in the end you'll have spent a life looking very good—but not living very well!

Remember, as Margaret Thatcher said, "Being powerful is like being a lady—if you have to tell people you are, you aren't."

NUMBER **1** **Plan big and dream greatness.**

As Nancy Astor said, The penalty of success is to be bored by the attentions of people who formerly snubbed you.

No person has the right to rain on your dreams.

And when the day arrives that you are on top of your game, thank God, and be kind to those who never believed in you because, after all, the best revenge is success.

* * *

My lifelong principle: service is the rent you pay for living, and that service is what sets you apart.

When duty calls, be prepared to answer.

Afterword

Nilda Morales, President and CEO, Society of Education and Rehabilitation of Puerto Rico

Dynamic, sensitive, and simple words are necessary to describe Dr. Antonia Coello Novello.

Her attributes, of vast experience and intelligence, are plenty and diverse and are reflected in the captivating sparkle of her eyes, with a deep, curious, and restless but equally accessible gaze, that inspires those around her with respect and trustworthiness, and a portion of good humor. That was the first impression we had when we first met her, which inspired us and has intensified over time due to her significant feats.

Visionary and passionate about life itself, she has been a consistent worldwide spokesperson for equity for all people. This path has been her motto, and she has translated it into providing essential services to the vulnerable and deprived populations of Puerto Rico in the most apprehensive and devastating moments following natural disasters or health emergencies, such as when the COVID-19 epidemic emerged. Her committed work has likewise extended to other Hispanic communities in the Caribbean as well as Central and South America through the partnership she maintains with international NGOs.

Novello was born in Fajardo, Puerto Rico, of humble origin, but with a solid foundation based in education and true values. Her character structure was instilled by her mother, a teacher for more than six decades in her hometown. Novello developed an extraordinarily strong personality with heart-driven vision and perseverance, a product of both her health challenges and the reality with which she had to deal and overcome all throughout her childhood and early adulthood when she was bullied and rejected due to her congenital physiological condition. It was these challenges that endowed her with an unbreakable will, self-esteem, and self-confidence that do not depend on external factors or praise but rather on the knowledge that her own internal power and transformative capacity were enough to pursue and achieve her dreams. Being very young, that self-determination catapulted her to positions never before held by women, and even less by Hispanics, positioned next to the main influential political leaders of the moment.

She has been recognized globally as a health leader, educator, humanitarian, and philanthropist, generously and willingly serving as a spokesperson for human rights and public policy changes that improve the lives of citizens, especially people with stigmatized conditions, such as AIDS, disabilities, or autism. As a pediatrician, she has altruistically designed and actively participated in educational programs for new parents on the proper developmental milestones of an infant's growth. The "Asi Debo Crecer" (As I Grow) program, bilingual, with a sixth-grade comprehension level, and for which she recorded videos, was made freely accessible to all parents of infants under two years of age, preventing gaps—sometimes imperceptible—that could affect the child's learning process or subsequent behavior.

Novello believes in inclusion and a world free of barriers, be they ideological, physical, attitudinal, or misconceptions, and to instead build spaces for the full development and access of all to education, health, food, housing, and protection. She believes in alliances between governments and nonprofit organizations to achieve relevant results where they are most needed and that transcend the moment and become longitudinal changes.

Her professional career has transpired in harmony with her personal beliefs. Those who know her know that she exemplifies that what is important in life is not who you are, but what you do and accomplish so that others may reach their full potential and resources. The responsibility, then, lies in developing a foundation where everyone can grow, learn, and build to meet the collective basic needs for a balanced, satisfying, and productive life. Dr. Antonia Novello, whose life story is inspiringly told in *Duty Calls*, is, without a doubt, a hero of our era.

Afterword

James J. Barba, JD, President Emeritus,
Albany Medical Center

To the best of my recollection, it was midmorning on the first Friday of September 1999 when my assistant rang the line that connected our offices. When I picked up, she said to me, "Jim, Dr. Antonia Novello, the new State Health Commissioner, is looking to speak with you. She's on the line." Since Dr. Novello had been on the job for about a month, she and I had yet to have the opportunity to meet or speak. Nonetheless, I asked that she be put through to me immediately. Her opening words were chilling: "Barba, you and I have a problem," she said. "I think that it's going to be a serious one."

The last month of the summer is an idyllic time in Upstate New York. The remaining days of August and the early September days, particularly before school opens, are warm enough for all outdoor activities, and the nights are cool enough to invite sleeping with the windows open. I live in northeastern New York, in Albany County, the state's capital, but the counties to the south—Columbia and Green—and those to the north—Saratoga, Warren, and Washington—are each unique and perfect at this time of year as well.

While Albany's business is government, the economies of most of its surrounding counties are centered on agriculture, and the farther one goes from Albany, the more agriculture predominates. At least that was the case at the end of the twentieth century.

The combination of the exceptional weather and the agricultural environment contributed to one of the region's special activities during each August—the county fair. County fairs combine the showing of residents' livestock and produce, and they usually have rides, games, and the like, all in a carnival atmosphere. They are fun for the entire family—particularly youngsters—at an affordable price. Many upstate counties sponsor these fairs, but among the most celebrated is the Washington County Fair, begun around 1840 and continued to this day. People come from the entire region to attend it.

In September of 1999, I was in my fifth year as President and CEO of the Albany Medical Center. Albany Med is one of the nation's approximately 130 academic medical centers, consisting of its own medical college, the region's only Children's Hospital—with the highest level Pediatric and Neonatal Intensive Care Units—the only level 1 Trauma Center, and many other clinical programs unique in northeastern New York. I was an unusual choice for the CEO position of such a complex medical constellation, since I am neither a physician nor a scientist. I am an attorney. Early in August of 1999, I had decided that I would not have time to attend the Washington County Fair that year. Little did I know that the fair would be coming to me.

Dr Antonia Novello was the 14th Surgeon General of the United States, serving in the role by appointment from President George H. W. Bush. In 1999, following her service as Surgeon General, New York State Governor George Pataki chose her as the state's Commissioner of Health. That position is among the most complex medical jobs in the nation, and Dr. Novello served in it with distinction until the end of Governor Pataki's final term as Governor in 2006. She lived through more genuine health crises (including the health issues arising from the attacks on 9/11) than can be recounted here. But that telephone call to me in September 1999 was to be her first.

On the phone, I can recall asking Dr. Novello what was happening. "Barba," she said, "I need to come to your office right away. My staff is telling me that we have a serious outbreak of *E. coli* from the Washington County Fair. I'll be in your office in fifteen minutes."

A couple of thoughts remain with me from this conversation. First, Dr. Novello called me "Barba" with no title before my name. I would learn later that this was the way she addressed many of her friends. Over the years that we worked together, she would call me "Barba," and I would call her "Commissioner."

Second, as soon as I hung up, I called our hospital's Medical Director. He told me that, in fact, we had a few patients being seen for *E. coli* infections—at that point they were children, and a couple of them were in serious condition. I informed him of my conversation with the Health Commissioner and suggested that he should get ready for an influx of patients, both children and adults.

When Dr. Novello arrived, her mood was completely composed, but tense. As a board-certified pediatrician (a pediatric nephrologist, in fact), her first thoughts were for the children who would be infected with *E. coli*. There was deep empathy as she explained that *E. coli* was more likely to be fatal to children than to adults; that infected children became very sick very quickly; that these children would have to be placed on a special form of dialysis immediately because the strain of *E. coli* that had been found released toxins into the blood stream that destroy the kidneys and then, quickly, brain tissue; and that children were more susceptible to this outcome because of their underdeveloped immune systems.

She asked if she could speak with our chief pediatric infectious disease physician right away as well as to the physician in charge of the entire Children's Hospital. She made it clear to me that we had to *move*, and that she would help us to do that.

Sometimes skill and luck coincide, and this was one of those times. Our chief pediatric infectious disease physician was Dr. Martha (Marty) Lepow. Marty had a national reputation as a leader in her field. Dr. Novello spoke with her at length, and they both agreed on two important factors: our Pediatric Intensive Care Unit (PICU) of seventeen beds was not large enough to handle the number of children who would need care, and we might need upwards of twenty pediatric hemodialysis machines. We had fewer than ten and had never needed to use all of them at one time.

The *E. coli* outbreak was traced by Dr. Novello's team to contaminated water from the Washington County Fair. That water started being used during the last few days of August. It took several days after exposure for the children and adults to show symptoms. So, the Friday I am referring to, and the following weekend, were critical days for many of those infected to go to local physicians or emergency rooms. As soon as that happened, and just as Dr Novello predicted, Albany Med saw a heavy inflow of patients.

That Friday, and the following two weeks, were a blur of activity. The Commissioner had a unique way of taking charge without appearing to override the authority of the Medical Center's physicians. As the state's chief public health regulator, she could immediately waive certain requirements for operating PICU beds. The waiver allowed us to convert adult beds into PICU beds to handle the overflow of critically ill children. She also had her staff call other Children's Hospitals in the state, asking to borrow some of their pediatric dialysis equipment. There was never a doubt in my mind that her quick, unflinching decisions during those early days helped save the lives of every child who came to us with *E. coli*, except for one. Her easy command also sent a similar message of urgency to the adult side of the hospital, and those physicians, too, were ready to care for a wave of adult patients.

Most of us can no longer recall a time before smart phones and social media, which allow the almost instantaneous transmission of news, both true and false. But 1999 was such a time, and Commissioner Novello recognized that reporting on the *E. coli* outbreak would occur both formally on news networks and by quickly spreading rumor, much of it erroneous. It was for this reason that, in addition to all the other things she asked me for, she wanted the use of an auditorium.

Again displaying great empathy, she told me that all parents and family members of the infected patients should have access to her, and to the treating physicians, so that they could be given timely and accurate information. She was right. Each day all parents and family were invited to our Huyck Auditorium at five p.m. There they were given complete information about where the crisis stood, how the children (and the adults) were doing, and what she saw as immediate next steps. She answered all questions frankly and in plain English. She told the parents, "I want you to hear these things from me, before you hear them on the six o'clock news." In this way, she won the hearts of those who were so desperately concerned about their kids and their family members. In a sense, she became her own "facebook" before Facebook.

The crisis lasted about three weeks. And, when it was over, more than twenty children, who had to be dialyzed because of the seriousness of their illness, survived and went home, as did many more who were not as critically ill. Moreover, all adults treated by Albany Med recovered. During those three weeks, Dr. Novello was everywhere throughout the hospital. Whether at three in the morning or three in the afternoon, she was in the PICU reassuring parents and talking with the children. Whether it was breakfast, lunch, or dinner, she was in our cafeteria making herself available to anyone who wanted to speak with her. Her constant presence assured, reassured, and calmed all who were involved, including many on the hospital staff. To me, it seemed that she never slept or rested.

As I have thought back over this time, I have tried to put my finger, precisely, on how to describe what it was that allowed Dr. Antonia Novello both to succeed in her mission to save the children and to develop the confidence of every person who worked with her.

Certainly, there was her clinical skill. There were her very apparent leadership qualities. There was her demonstrated empathy. There was her reputation as an outstanding Surgeon General. All of these helped. But together they don't capture what was at the heart of her work that September. What does capture it is much simpler. Despite all her titles and her professional successes, Dr. Novello truly loved the children, and she adopted the role as a type of "mother-in-chief." She was completely determined to move heaven and earth to save all of them. And, against heavy odds, save them is exactly what she did.

In the six years that followed, it was my privilege to work with this outstanding physician whose life story is told in *Duty Calls*. Usually, we agreed on how to solve our problems. Sometimes we disagreed. But we worked through every one of them successfully . . . with me as "Barba" and Dr. Novello as "Commissioner."

Acknowledgments

We would like to thank the tremendous personnel at Fulcrum for their support of this project and their faith in us. Especially Sam Scinta, Kateri Kramer, Alison Auch, and Patty Maher.

Toni: I want to acknowledge so many friends—old ones and new ones—who have been instrumental in my life. So many to mention, but I want to acknowledge in particular my colleagues who wrote the forewords, afterwords, and endorsements. They have a special place in my heart. My life's gratitude and also my respect for the Surgeons General, and my godchildren: Diego, Santi, and Cisco. Also Lydia, Yolly, Linette, General Reyes, General Buchanan, General Ramirez, Lisa, Michael and Marcia, Rosa Bell, Elena Crosby, Marife, Salvi, Maria Fernanda, David, Enery, Ricardo, Yazmin, Emanuel, Nancy, Diana, Charlie G., Joyce, Ken R., Carolina, Ana Gloria, Luisa, Saul, J. B., Josefina, Marta, Toñito, Gustavo, the Ariza family and Guillermo, Carmen, Juan, Gabi, Nilda, Aidita, Luis, Iche, Stephy, Tito, Ferdinand, Wilma, Rita, Idalina, Myrna, Ivette, Aida, Edaliz, Graciela, Ina, Luz, Norma, Anna, Evelyn, Chanie S., Marissa, Chica, Tulio, Nathan, the Arraiza family, E. Stewart Jones, Franklin, Ken, Marlena, Jorge, PACIV, Lili and Jivanny, Dean Compton, and, of course, my whole family: Mama, Mami Loli, Tomas, Mayra, Mayte, Tanya, Monin, Ivonne, and Joe's family, Eileen, and Don. And my medical classes of 1969 and 1970 from Puerto Rico. To the doctors at the Mayo Clinic, Dr. Quinones-Hinojosa, Dr. Juan Canabal, Dr. Carlos Pérez-Vega, and Kojo. And all the employees of the Hyatt House San Juan who cared for me for the last six years while I assisted with the Puerto Rico recovery. I apologize in advance for any omissions.

Toni: To the Naval Captain at Bethesda Naval Hospital who did not interview me for a job. I owe him the largest part of my success. His actions prompted me to join the US Public Health Service at the National Institutes of Health instead of securing a naval post at Bethesda. That made all the difference—and the rest is history.

Toni: To Jill, my co-author, who gave me the opportunity to write my book, who motivated me, who found us the publisher, and who was able to put into words my life as I would have written it.

Jill: To Gail Berkey and Ann Kellan whose review of the drafts was invaluable.

To Jill's village, who support her through thick and thin, including through her divorce, which happened during the writing and production of this book.

Awards and Honors

—HONORS—

1970 Graduated top 5% of Puerto Rico School of Medicine, San Juan, PR

1971 Intern of the Year Award, University of Michigan, Dept. of Pediatrics, Ann Arbor, MI

1987 Member, Society for Pediatric Research

1987 Member, The American Pediatric Society

1987 Member, Alpha Omega Alpha Medical Society

1990 American Medical Women Association Leadership Award, Philadelphia, PA

1991 Medical Center Alumni Society Award, University of Michigan, Ann Arbor, MI

1991 The Woodrow Wilson Award for Distinguished Government Service, Johns Hopkins University, Alumni Assoc., Baltimore, MD

1991 The Johns Hopkins University Society of Scholars, Baltimore, MD

1991 The Elizabeth Blackwell Medal, Hobart and William Smith College, Wash., DC

1992 Charles C. Shepard Science Award for Scientific Excellence, Wash., DC

1992 Health Leader Award, Commissioned Officers Association, UPHS, Cincinnati, OH

1992 National Council of La Raza—President's Award, Los Angeles, CA

1993 American Medical Association, Nathan Davis Award, Chicago, IL

1993 American Academy of Pediatrics, Excellence in Public Service Award, Wash., DC

1993 Member, Delta Omega Public Health Honorary Society, Alpha Chapter, Baltimore, MD

1993 University of Michigan Alumni Council Athena Award, Ann Arbor, MI

1993 American Medical Association Board of Trustees Special Award for Meritorious Service, Chicago, IL

1994 Induction, National Women's Hall of Fame, Seneca Falls, NY

1994 Healthy American Fitness Award, Palm Springs, CA

1995 Ronald McDonald Children's Charities Award of Excellence, Chicago, IL

1996 Miami Children's Hospital International Pediatric Hall of Fame, Miami, FL

1997 Distinguished Alumni Award, American Association of State Colleges and Universities, Wash., DC

1998 Dean's Medal, The Johns Hopkins School of Hygiene & Public Health, Baltimore, MD

1998 Hispanic Heritage Awards—Leadership Award, Kennedy Center, Wash., DC

1999 COSSMHO—Hispanic Health Leadership Award—Humanitarian Award for Lifetime Achievement, Wash., DC

2000 Member, Institute of Medicine of the National Academy of Sciences, Wash., DC

2000 Luther L. Terry Award for Exemplary Leadership in Tobacco Control, Chicago, IL

2000 NIH Office of Research on Minority Health Distinguished Service Award for Contributions Towards Reducing/Eliminating Racial Health Disparities, Wash., DC

2001 American Cancer Society Humanitarian Award, New York, NY

2001 David B. Kriser Medallion—NYU College of Dentistry, New York, NY

2002 University Medal of Honor, State University of NY at Stony Brook, NY

2002 American Medical Women's Assoc. International Women in Medicine Hall of Fame, Wash., DC

2002 Dean's Distinguished Service Award, Mailman School of Public Health, Columbia University, New York, NY

2002 Smithsonian Institute, The James Smithson Bicentennial Medal, Wash., DC

2002   Baruch College—City University New York President's Medal, New York, NY

2003   The Face of Medicine, Achievements of Women in Medicine Exhibition, National Library of Medicine, Bethesda, MD

2004   Portraits of Latino Achievements Exhibition, Our Journeys/Our Stories, Smithsonian's National Museum of American History, Wash., DC

2005   National Governor's Association Distinguished Service to State Government Award, Des Moines, Iowa

2006   Ethel Le Frak Award, National Osteoporosis Foundation, New York, NY

2006   Helen Rodriguez-Trias AIDS Institute Award, NY Dept. of Health, Albany, NY

2007   Latina of Excellence Award, *Hispanic Magazine*, New York, NY

2008   Legacy Award for Sciences, Smithsonian Institute Latino Center, Washington, DC

2009   Coquí de Oro Award—Casa de Puerto Rico, Orlando, FL

2011   El Quixote Award for Lifetime Achievement, Orlando, FL

2013   Women Who Mean Business, *Orlando Business Journal*, Orlando, FL

2013   Women of Distinction, Lifetime Achievement Award, Girl Scouts of Citrus Council, Orlando, FL

2017   Martin Luther King, Jr. Keynote Speaker, University of Pennsylvania School of Medicine, Philadelphia, PA

2017   10th Annual Domenici Conference—Keynote Speaker—NMU—Las Cruces, NM

—VISITING LECTURESHIPS—

1991   50th Anniversary of the University of Michigan, School of Public Health, "A Vision for Health in the 21st Century," Ann Arbor, MI, Sept.

1995   George Armstrong Lecture, Ambulatory Pediatric Association, "The State of the World's Children," Ambulatory Pediatric Association, San Diego, CA, May

1995   Dr. Emilio Soto Annual Lectureship, "Health Care Challenges for the Year 2000," Northern Virginia Pediatric Society, McLean, VA, Sept.

1995 Amberg Hemholtz Lectureship—22nd Mayo Clinic Pediatric Days, "The Needs of Children in the Political Reality of Today," Mayo Foundation, Rochester, MN, Sept.

1996 The A. Clifford Barger Hinton-Wright Lecture, "The Future of Minorities in Health Care Reform," Harvard Medical School, Boston, MA, May

1996 Second Annual Endowed Philip Kozinn Visiting Professorship, "Changing the World of Our Children and Their Health," Maimonides Medical Center, Brooklyn, NY, Oct.

1998 Forum 98: 150th Anniversary of the Seneca Falls Convention, "Long-Term Care—A Woman's Dilemma," Elizabeth Blackwell Institute—Susan B. Anthony Center, University of Rochester, Rochester, NY, July

1998 Santiago Ramón y Cajal Memorial Lecture, "Latinos—The Emerging Majority—Who Are We? And Where Are We Going?" XXII Inter-American Medical Congress, New York, NY

1999 The First Annual Dr. Leroy Burney Lecture, "The Health of the Nation: A Century in Perspective," Johns Hopkins University, School of Hygiene and Public Health, Baltimore, MD, July

2000 Theobald Smith Lecture Award, "The Art of Medicine—Quo Vadis?" Albany Medical College, Albany, NY

2000 Charles Elwood Memorial Lecture, "Public Health in NY: A Microcosm of The World," Buffalo Academy of Medicine, Buffalo, NY, May

2001 Dr. Bryant L. Galusha Lecture, "Today's Vision—Tomorrow's Reality," Federation State Medical Boards, Atlanta, GA

2001 17th Annual James Earle Ash Lecture, "The Modern Era Surgeon General—A Retrospective Review," Armed Forces Institute of Pathology, Wash., DC

2002 14th Annual NICHD-NIH Maternal-Fetal-Neonatal Reproductive Medicine: Butterfield Memorial Lecture, "Bioterrorism—Preparedness and Lessons Learned," Aspen, CO, Aug.

2004 Stockton Kimbal Lecture, "Medicine—Professionalism and Ethics," Medical Alumni Association, University of Buffalo School of Medicine and Biomedical Sciences, Roswell Park Cancer Institute, Buffalo, NY, May

2005 The Donald A. Berreth Lecture, "Headlines and Lifelines: The Role of Public Health Information Before, During and After Disaster," Atlanta, GA, Oct.

2018 Primary Care Conference of the US Armed Forces—Primary Care Today—Jacksonville, FL, March

2022 Keynote Speaker, Nathan F. Mossell Lecture, University of Pennsylvania, Philadelphia, PA

2022 BDHEA Summit—Surgeons General Panel, Health Equity Today

—UNIFORMED SERVICES AWARDS—

1983 USPHS Commendation Medal
1983 USPHS Special Assignment Service Ribbon
1984 USPHS Citation Award
1984 USPHS Exceptional Capacity Promotion to Captain
1987 USPHS Regular Corps Ribbon
1988 USPHS Unit Commendation
1988 USPHS Outstanding Service Medal
1989 USPHS Surgeon General's Exemplary Service Medal
1989 DHHS Assistant Secretary for Health Certificate of Commendation
1989 USPHS Outstanding Unit Citation
1990 USPHS Unit Commendation
1990 USPHS Foreign Duty Service Ribbon
1990 USPHS Meritorious Service Medal
1990 USPHS Achievement Medal
1990 USPHS Surgeon General's Medallion
1990 USPHS National Emergency Preparedness Ribbon
1990 US Army Commander's Award for Public Service
1991 USPHS Chief Nurse Officer's Award
1992 USPHS Unit Commendation
1992 The Association of Military Surgeons of the US Founders Medal
1992 United States Coast Guard Meritorious Service Medal
1992 USPHS Distinguished Service Medal
1992 Order of Military Medical Merit, US Army

1992   USPHS Crisis Response Service Award

1993   USPHS Chief Nurse Officer's Award

1993   The Under Secretary for Health Award, Dept. of Veterans Affairs

1993   Department of Defense, Legion of Merit Medal, US Army

1993   Department of the Air Force Exceptional Civilian Service Award

1993   Bronze Medal for Commendable Service, US Environmental Protection Agency

1993   Department of the Navy Distinguished Public Service Award

1994   USPHS Unit Commendation

1995   Veterans of Foreign Wars James E. Van Zandt Citizenship Award

1998   Bicentennial Unit Commendation

1999   USPHS Distinguished Service Medal

2018   Global Health Campaign Medal

2018   Humanitarian Service Medal, US Army, USPHS

2018   Unit Citation for Puerto Recovery During Hurricane Maria, USPHS

2018   Jones Act Centennial Medal of US Citizenship, Government of Puerto Rico, San Juan, Department of State

2018   Civilian Award for Humanitarian Service, United States Army North (Fifth Army), Department of the Army Fort Sam Houston, Texas

2018   Distinguished Service Medal for Extraordinary Professional Commitment During the Aftermath of Maria, Military Forces of Puerto Rico and Governor of Puerto Rico

2019   Meritorious Public Service Medal for Exceptional Service during the Recovery Operations in Puerto Rico during Hurricane Maria, United States Army North, Department of the Army

2023   Puerto Rico National Guard, Merit Cross Medal

—AWARDS AND OTHER SELECTED RECOGNITIONS—

1980   Woman of the Year Award—Distinguished Graduates Public School System, San Juan, PR

1985   *Who's Who in the South and Southwest*—19th ed.

1985   Certificate of Recognition—Employees Advisory Committee, DRG, NIH

1987–Pres.   *Who's Who in America*

1987   Certificate of Recognition, Distinguished Alumni, Medical Sciences Campus, University of Puerto Rico, San Juan

1987–Pres.   *Who's Who of American Women*

1988, 1992   *American Men and Women of Science*

1988   Achievement Award, National Conference of Puerto Rican Women, Miami

1989   US Delegate to President Mitterrand's First Meeting of the International Ethics Committee on AIDS, Paris, France

1990   First Recipient of El Premio al Servicio Público, Fundación Felisa Rincón De Gautier, San Juan, PR

1990   Life Achievement Award, The National Puerto Rican Coalition, Wash., DC

1990   Georgeanna Seeger Jones Award, American Fertility Assoc., Wash., DC

1990   Ronald McDonald Children's Charities of Puerto Rico, Premio Excelencia, San Juan, PR

1990   Woman of Achievement Award, Texas Woman's University, Dallas, TX

1990   The Woman of Leadership Award, University of Michigan, Ann Arbor

1990   Lillian D. Wald Award, New York, NY

1990   Award for Service to Humanity, Puerto Rican Chamber of Commerce in the United States, NY

1990   Las Primeras Award, Mexican American Women's National Association, Wash., DC

1990   National Institutes of Health—Directors Award, Bethesda, MD

1991   Living Legacy Award, Women's International Center, San Diego, CA

1991   Medical Achievement Award, American Liver Foundation, Wash., DC

1991   Puerto Rican Family Institute Award, New York, NY

1991   Premio a la Excelencia, Escuela de Odontología, San Juan, PR

1991   Outstanding Achievement Award, National Association of Cuban American Women, Wash., DC

1991   Congressional Hispanic Caucus Medal, Wash., DC

1991   National Osteoporosis Foundation Award, Wash., DC

1991   Simon Bolivar, National Award Recipient, New York, NY

1991   National Association of Community Health Centers Leadership Award, San Francisco, CA

1991   Juan Carlos Finlay Award for Leadership, Hispanic Officers Steering Committee, USPHS, Rockville, MD

1991   *Who's Who Among Hispanic Americans*

1992   American Association of Women Emergency Physicians and American College of Emergency Physicians Health Policy Section Award, Wash., DC

1992   National Leadership Award, Wash., DC

1992   The *Washington Times* Freedom Award, Wash., DC

1992   Roberto Clemente Humanitarian Award, Boricua College, New York, NY

1992   Saving Lives Coalition Certificate of Appreciation, Wash., DC

1992   "The Golden Plate Award," American Academy of Achievement, Las Vegas, NV

1992   The George Crile Award, International Platform Assoc., Wash., DC

1992   Government Leaders Against Drunk Driving (Gladd Award), Orlando, FL

1992   Outstanding Service Award in the Field of Medical Services, CCM of East Los Angeles College, Los Angeles, CA

1992   Dean's Appreciation Award, The Johns Hopkins University School of Hygiene and Public Health, Baltimore, MD

1992   Elizabeth Ann Seton Award, National Catholic Education Association, Wash., DC

1992   National Conference of Puerto Rican Women Award, New York, NY

1992   National Council on Alcoholism and Drug Dependence, Gold Key Award, Wash., DC

1992   Mother Gerard Phelan Gold Medal Award, Marymount University, Arlington, VA

1992   Massachusetts Drug Fighters of the Year Award, Governor's Alliance Against Drugs, Dorchester, MA

1992   American Association for Marriage and Family Therapy, Distinguished Leadership Award, Miami, FL

1992   Stop Teenage Addiction to Tobacco (STAT) Leadership Award, San Francisco, CA

1993   La Leche League International Award of Recognition, Wash., DC

1993   Outstanding Achievements in Early Childhood Immunization Award, DHHS, Wash., DC

1993   Ellis Island Congressional Medal of Honor, Ellis Island, NY

1993   Western Hemispheric Conference on Persons with Disabilities Award, Wash., DC

1993   Woman of Distinction Award, Wash., DC

1993   Paul Harris Fellow Award, Rotary Foundation of Rotary International, San Juan, PR

1993   Women of Achievement, Beyond the Glass Ceiling Award, New York

1993   Florette Pomeroy Award, Women's Alcoholism Center, San Francisco, CA

1993   Puerto Rican AIDS Foundation Award, San Juan, PR

1993   The National Citation Award—Mortar Board Inc., Wash., DC

1994   Public Leadership Education Network Mentor Award, Wash., DC

1994   Hispanic Elected Local Officials Distinguished Service Award Wash., DC

1994   Mount Sinai Medical Center Community Service Award, New York, NY

1994   *Hispanic Magazine* Award for Lifetime Achievement, Wash., DC

1994   "Si, Se Puede Award," PHS Hispanic Heritage Month, Capitol Hill, Wash., DC

1995   Union of American Women, Premio Monumento a la Mujer, Ponce, PR

1995   GALA 12 Birmingham-Southern College Award, Birmingham, AL

1995   Coqui de Oro—Union of American Women, Puerto Rico Chapter, San Juan, PR

1995   National Council of Catholic Women/Distinguished Service Award, San Francisco, CA

1996   General Fernando Chardon Award, San Juan, PR

1996   Jose Celso Barbosa Health Award, National Puerto Rican Parade, New York, NY

1996   Women at Work Science Award, Wash., DC

1996   Hispanic Hero Award, 15th Annual US Hispanic Leadership Conf., Chicago, IL

1996   Premio Extraordinario, Instituto de Puerto Rico, New York, NY

1996   Georgetown University Vicennial Medal—for Loyal Distinguished Service, Wash., DC

1998   Elena Mederos Award, National Association of Cuban American Women, Newark, NJ

1998   National Hispanic Heritage Foundation Award for Leadership, Wash., DC

1998   Mujer Award, The National Hispana Leadership Institute, Wash., DC

1998   Mayo Clinic and Mayo Foundation Women in Medicine Exhibit

1999   Charles R. Drew—Health Professional Humanitarian Award, Wash., DC

1999   New Horizon Award—National Association of Negro Business and Professional Women's Club, Inc., New York

1999   NYS Hispanic Heritage Committee Award, Hudson Valley Community College, NY

1999   Comité Noviembre Mes de la Herencia Puertorriqueña Award, New York, NY

2000   La Unidad Latina Distinguished Service Award, Brooklyn, NY

2000   National Coalition for Cancer Survivorship, National Public Leadership Award, Wash., DC

2000   YWCA Racial Justice Award, Wash., DC

2000   Cuban American National Council Public Service Award, Wash., DC

2000   Annual Mother's Day Tribute to Puerto Rican Women Award, New York, NY

2000   First Ladies Salute to Women Honoree, National First Ladies' Library, Smithsonian Museum of American History, Wash., DC

2000   Women in Excellence Award, Capital District Women's Business Council, Albany, NY

2000   Lifetime Achievement Award—Hispanic Business Roundtable Policy Conference, Temple University, Philadelphia, PA

2000   Latino Gerontological Center, Eighth Annual Golden Age Award, New York, NY

2000   New York State Federation of Hispanic Chambers of Commerce Outstanding Service Award, New York, NY

2000 New York State Nurses Association Presidential Award, Niagara, NY

2000 Leadership Award, National Hispanic Medical Association, New York, NY

2000 Outstanding Hispanic American Award, Long Island Chamber of Commerce, New York, NY

2000 Randolph Guggenheimer Public Service Award, New York, NY

2000 Lifetime Achievement Award, National Puerto Rican Coalition, Wash., DC

2000 Community Service Award, Institute for the Puerto Rican/Hispanic Elderly, New York, NY

2000 Ribbon of Hope Award, National Cancer Coalition Cancer Survivorship, Wash., DC

2000 Outstanding Leadership and Commitment to Improving the Lives of Individuals with Brain Injury and Their Families, Brain Injury Association of New York State, Schenectady, NY

2000 Excellence in Public Health Service Award, Latino Caucus, APHA, NY

2001 Community Service Award for Leadership and Support to Hispanic Women, Bronx, NY

2001 Career Achievements in the Health Field, Institute for the Puerto Rican/Hispanic Elderly, New York, NY

2001 100 Hispanic Women's Luminary Award, New York, NY

2001 88th Annual Chamber of Commerce Special Recognition Award, Puerto Rico Chamber of Commerce, Fajardo, PR

2001 2001 Public Health Leadership Award, NYS Public Health Association, Albany, NY

2001 Third Annual Advocacy Day of the Steering Committee of the Coalition for School-Based Primary Care, Albany, NY

2001 Helen Hayes MacArthur Award, Helen Hayes Hospital, NY

2001 Outstanding Service Award, National Stop the Violence Alliance, Inc., NY

2001 2001 Speaking Out for Justice Award, AAUW Legal Advocacy Fund, Austin, TX

2001 Distinguished Ex-Student Award, Universidad de Puerto Rico, San Juan, PR

2001 2001 St. Benedict Award, Benedictine Health Foundation, New Paltz, NY

2002 Distinguished Healthcare Advocate Award, Howard University Hospital, Wash., DC

2002 Ruby Slipper Award, "Sick Kids Need Involved People," New York, NY

2002 Entre Nosotras Award, Women's Caucus of the Puerto Rican/Hispanic Task Force, Albany, NY

2002 First Annual VISIONS for Latinos Award, Brooklyn Unidos, Brooklyn, NY

2002 The Women's Press Club of NYS 2002 Woman in the News Award, Albany, NY

2002 Avon Foundation Breast Cancer Crusade's Award, New York, NY

2002 The Helen Rodriguez-Trias Award, Latino Health: A Call to Action, NYU School of Medicine, New York, NY

2002 The National Medical Fellowship Lifetime Achievement Award, New York, NY

2002 New York-Presbyterian Healthcare System Award of Appreciation, White Plains, NY

2003 The 2003 Office Depot Visionary Award, Boca Raton, FL

2003 The Distinguished Service to the Nation's Public Health Award, San Antonio, TX

2003 Homeland Security Award—National Foundation for Women Legislators, Wash., DC

2003 The Prestigious Innovator Role Model Award, Minority Access, Inc., Wash., DC

2003 The Person of the Year Award, The Metropolitan Foundation, New York, NY

2003 The Community Commitment Award, Cobble Hill Health Center, Brooklyn, NY

2003 The Resource Woman Award, YWCA of Troy-Cohoes, Troy, NY

2004 Mujer a Todo Corazón—Cardiologist Association of Puerto Rico, San Juan, PR

2004 First Annual Reality Check Partner Award, Saratoga Springs, NY

2004 Museum of Science and Industry Board of Directors 2004 National Hispanic Scientist of the Year Award, Tampa, FL

2004 Vivian Pinn Distinguished Lecturer's Award, University of Virginia, Charlottesville, VA

2005 Distinguished Woman in the Field of Medicine and Personal Development Award, Women of the Americas Union, Ponce, PR

2006 "20 Rays of Hope," National Coalition for Cancer Survivorship, Wash., DC

2006 Women of the Américas Award, Unión de Mujeres de Las Américas, Inc., San Juan, PR

2006 Helen Manzer Award, College of Nursing, New York University, New York, NY

2006 Helen Rodriguez-Trias AIDS Institute Award, New York State Department of Health, Albany, NY

2007 Latina of Excellence Award, *Hispanic Magazine*, New York, NY

2013 "50 Women Who Shaped America's Health," *Huffington Post*, New York, NY

2013 Women Who Mean Business Award, Orlando Business Journal, Orlando, FL

2013 Lifetime Achievement, Women of Distinction Awards, Orlando, FL

2014 Public Health Hero, Florida Department of Health, Orange County, FL

2015 Meritorious Service as Surgeon General, National Medical Association, Detroit, MI

2015 Recognition Award, Diversity Speakers, Philadelphia College of Osteopathic Medicine, Philadelphia, PA

2016 Appreciation Award, Hispanic Women Chamber of Commerce, Orlando, FL

2016 Distinction Award, Feinberg School of Medicine, Office of Diversity and Inclusion, Lyceum Series, Chicago, IL

2017 Latino Excellence Award, Salem State University, Latin American Student Organization, Salem, MA

2017 Honorary Citation, The Commonwealth of Massachusetts, House of Representatives, Boston, MA

2017   Excellence in Crisis and Risk Communication Award, University of Central Florida, Orlando, FL

2017   LASO—Latin American Student Organization, Latino Excellence Award, Latinos Connection Conference—Salem, MA

2017   Mocion Reconocimiento Y Agradecimiento—Huracan Maria Camara De Representantes—Capitolio Puerto Rico, San Juan, PR

2017   Support Award, A Night with Nemours, Nemours Hospital for Children, Orlando, FL

2017   Women in Medicine Award, University of Pennsylvania, Philadelphia, PA

2017   Government of Puerto Rico Recognition Award for Services Rendered During Hurricane Maria, Government of Puerto Rico House of Representatives, San Juan, PR

2018   Government of Puerto Rico Recognition Award, House of Representatives, Puerto Rico Capital, San Juan, PR

2018   Recognition Award for Excellent Performance During Hurricane Maria, Puerto Rico Secretary of Health Award, Department of Health, San Juan, PR

2018   Recognition Award, Women's Month, Government of Puerto Rico House of Representatives, San Juan, PR

2018   Department of Health Puerto Rico Award for Collaborating During Hurricane Maria, Department of Health Puerto Rico, San Juan, PR

2018   Conversatorio Mujer—Diferentes Miradas Camara Representantes—P.R. CapitolioMocion de Agradecimiento, Mes De La Mujer, Ponce, PR

2018   Dolores C. Huerta Woman of Courage Medallion, United States Hispanic Leadership Institute, Chicago, Illinois

2018   The San Felipe Del Morro Award, Puerto Rico Alliance of Florida, Nuestro Futuro Symposium—FIU, Miami, FL

2018   Impact Leader for Advocacy, Change Maker Impact Awards, United Way, Heart of Florida, Orlando, FL

2018   Special Recognition Award, Teachers Association of Puerto Rico, Annual Assembly, San Juan, PR

2018   Lifetime Hispanic Achievers Award, Orlando Museum of Art, Orlando, FL

2018   Hispanic Public Health Conference, CHISPA Award for Starting the Applied Knowledge for the Health of the Puerto Rican People, Awarded by Former Secretary of Health, Puerto Rico, San Juan, PR

2019   Woman Who Leads Award, Womanpreneur, San Juan, PR

2019   Immunization Award of Excellence, VOCES, San Juan, PR

2019   Congratulation Award during International Women's Month, Government of Puerto Rico Senate, San Juan, PR

2020   Service Award, University of Michigan Frankel Cardiovascular Center, Ann Arbor, MI

2020   Named in *USA TODAY*'s 100 Women of the Century, Women in Science, Medicine and Education

2020   Featured in the book, *100 American Women Who Changed the World*, Publications International

2020   Lifetime Achievement Award, 26th Anniversary, *Latina Style Magazine*, Orlando, FL

2021   Premio a la Excelencia del Servicio al Projimo, Sister Isolina Ferré Award, House of Representatives, San Juan, PR

2022   Diamond Award, Heroes COVID 19, VOCES, San Juan, PR

2022   Office of Diversity, Inclusion and Community Engagement, Module Renaming Honoree, Oklahoma Medical School, Oklahoma City, OK

—HONORARY DEGREES—

1990   Honorary Doctor of Science, Medical College of Ohio, Toledo, OH

1990   Honorary Doctor of Science, Universidad Central del Caribe, Cayey, PR

1990   Honorary Doctor of Law Degree, College of Notre Dame of Maryland, Baltimore, MD

1990   Honorary Doctor Humane Letters, Meharry Medical College, Nashville, TN

1991   Honorary Doctor of Science Degree, University of Notre Dame, South Bend, IN

1991   Distinguished Visiting Professor, Marymount University, Arlington, VA

1992   Honorary Doctor of Science, Lehigh University, Bethlehem, PA

1992   Honorary Doctor of Science, Hood College, Frederick, MD

1992   Honorary Doctor of Public Health, Providence College, Providence, RI

1992   Honorary Doctor of Science, New York Medical College, Valhalla, NY

1992   Honorary Doctor of Public Service, Washington and Jefferson College, Washington, PA

1992   Honorary Doctor of Science, University of Massachusetts, Worcester, MA

1992   Honorary Doctor of Science, Florida International University, Miami, FL

1993   Honorary Doctor of Science, Washington College, Chestertown, MD

1993   Honorary Doctor of Law Degree, American University, Wash., DC

1993   Honorary Doctor of Science, Catholic University, Wash., DC

1993   Honorary Doctor of Science, Saint Mary's College, South Bend, IN

1993   Honorary Doctor of Humane Letters, State University of New York, Farmingdale, NY

1993   Honorary Doctor of Science, Eastern Virginia Medical School, Norfolk, VA

1993   Honorary Doctor of Humane Letters, Mount St. Mary's College, Emmitsburg, MD

1993   Honorary Doctor of Science, Central Connecticut State University, New Britain, CT

1993   Honorary Doctorate of Science, Georgetown University, Washington, DC

1993   Honorary Doctor of Humane Letters, La Salle University, Philadelphia, PA

1994   Honorary Doctor of Law, University of Michigan, Ann Arbor, MI

1995   Honorary Doctor of Public Service, University of Portland, Portland, OR

1995   Honorary Doctor of Humane Letters, NY College of Osteopathic Medicine, Westbury, NY

1995   Honorary Doctor of Humane Letters, Mount Sinai School of Medicine, New York, NY

1996   Honorary Doctor of Humane Letters, Alvernia College, Reading, PA

1996 Honorary Doctorate of Humanities, King's College, Wilkes-Barre, PA

1996 Honorary Doctorate of Health Sciences, Ponce School of Medicine, PR

1997 Honorary Doctor of Law, Gannon University, Erie, PA

1997 Honorary Doctor of Humane Letters, Loyola University, Chicago, IL

1998 Honorary Doctor of Humane Letters and Science, Caribbean University, San Juan, PR

2000 Honorary Doctor of Science, D'Youville College, Buffalo, NY

2000 Honorary Doctor of Science, Montclair State University, East Rutherford, NJ

2000 Honorary Doctor of Public Service, Russell Sage College, Troy, NY

2001 Honorary Doctor of Science, School of Medicine and Dentistry, University of Rochester, NY

2002 Honorary Doctor of Public Service, University of North Texas, Fort Worth, TX

2002 Honorary Doctor of Science, Albany College of Pharmacy, Albany, NY

2003 Honorary Doctor of Science, Universidad Autónoma de Guadalajara, Guadalajara, México

2003 Honorary Doctor of Science, Howard University, Wash., DC

2003 Honorary Associate in Arts, Broward Community College, Fort Lauderdale, FL

2003 Honorary Doctor of Science, Pine Manor College, Chestnut Hill, MA

2003 Honorary Doctor of Science, New York University, New York, NY

2003 Honorary Doctor of Science, PACE University, New York, NY

2003 Honorary Doctor of Science, The College of New Rochelle, New Rochelle, NY

2003 Honorary Doctor in Arts, American University, Bayamon, PR

2004 Honorary Doctor of Humane Letters, College of Saint Rose, Albany, NY

2004 Honorary Doctor of Science, New York College of Osteopathic Medicine of New York Institute of Technology, Old Westbury, NY

2005 Honorary Doctor of Science, Chatham College, Pittsburgh, PA

2005 Honorary Doctor of Humane Letters, Charles R. Drew University School of Medicine, Los Angeles, CA

2006   Honorary Doctor of Humane Letters, Seton Hall University, South
       Orange, NJ
2007   Honorary Doctor of Humane Letters, NOVA Southeastern Univer-
       sity, Sunrise, FL
2013   Honorary Doctor of Humane Letters, Florida Technical College,
       Orlando, FL
2016   Honorary Doctor of Laws, Honoris Causa, Wayne State University
       School of Medicine, Detroit, MI
2017   Honorary Doctor of Humane Letters, Honoris Causa, Salem State
       University, Salem, MA
2020   Doctor of Public Health, Honoris Causa, San Juan Bautista School of
       Medicine, San Juan, PR
2022   Doctorate Honoris Causa in Humanities, San Juan Bautista School
       of Medicine, San Juan, PR

—NATIONAL SOCIETIES—

1975   American Academy of Pediatrics (Fellow)
1976   Latin American Society of Nephrology
1976   American Society of Nephrology
1978   International Society of Nephrology
1978   District of Columbia Medical Society (Associate Member)
1979   Pan American Medical and Dental Society
1980   The American Society of Pediatric Nephrology
1985   Association of Military Surgeons of the United States
1987   Society for Pediatric Research
1987   The American Pediatric Society
1987   Alpha Omega Alpha Medical Society
1990   Reserve Officers Association
1993   Delta Omega Honorary Public Health Society—Alpha Chapter
2000   The New York Academy of Medicine
2000   National Academy of Medicine
2001   Health Care Executive Forum

Discussion Questions

1. Does it surprise you that Dr. Novello has faced obstacles— some of them quite extreme—in her life? Why or why not?

2. Has there been an obstacle in your life that has been what you would call a "life-defining" event? How did you handle it?

3. Will the understanding that all of us face challenges help you go about your daily living? How? Why?

4. What themes for success have you adopted to date in your life?

5. Can you think of people in your life who have faced significant challenges? How did they overcome those challenges?

6. What kinds of challenges did Dr. Novello have in her life based on her being both a woman and Puerto Rican? How did she handle them? Give some examples.

7. What do you think is meant by "preparation meets opportunity equals success"? Are there examples from your own life where this formula has worked?

8. How do you think Dr. Novello's congenital megacolon helped shape her life?

9. Which of Dr. Novello's "Life Lessons" have worked for you in the past? Which do you see yourself applying in the future?

10. Some people consign older people to irrelevance. What can Dr. Novello's long life of service teach us about that attitude?

About the Authors

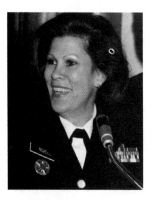

Dr. Antonia Coello Novello, 14th Surgeon General of the United States, was born in Fajardo, Puerto Rico. She graduated from the University of Puerto Rico with a BS degree in 1965 and an MD degree in 1970. She completed her pediatric internship and residency training in pediatrics at the University of Michigan, Ann Arbor, and a subspecialty fellowship in pediatric and adult nephrology at Georgetown University, and at the University of Michigan. In 1982, Dr. Novello received a master's degree in public health, and in May 2000 a doctorate in public health, both from Johns Hopkins University.

Dr. Novello is a member of the Alpha Omega Alpha Medical Society and a member of the National Academy of Medicine. She also belongs to the Johns Hopkins University Society of Scholars and is a member of the Delta Omega Public Health Honorary Society's Alpha chapter. She spent most of her professional career at the National Institutes of Health, where in 1986 she became Deputy Director of the National Institute of Child Health and Human Development.

On March 9, 1990, Dr. Novello was sworn in by Supreme Court Justice Sandra Day O'Connor to serve as the 14th Surgeon General of the US Public Health Service. Her appointment marked two firsts:

Dr. Novello became the first woman and the first Hispanic ever to hold this position, as well as the first career public health officer to become US Surgeon General in the recent past.

On June 3, 1999, Governor George E. Pataki nominated Dr. Novello to be the 13th New York State Health Commissioner; one of the leading health agencies in the nation with an annual budget of $49 billion. Most recently, Dr. Novello served as Vice President for Women and Children, and Executive Director of Public Health Policy at Florida Hospital. During that time, she was invited by the US ambassador to serve as a liaison between the government of the Dominican Republic and its Attorney General to raise awareness of domestic violence and was able to spearhead efforts that changed the previous national legislation.

During the COVID-19 pandemic, she became the spokesperson, public health advocate, and the provider and administrator of vaccines for all those in need in Puerto Rico. For her actions she received the Civilian Award for Humanitarian Service from the US Army, and the National Guard Merit Cross Medal.

Dr. Novello holds countless awards, among them the 1971 Department of Pediatrics—University of Michigan—Intern of the Year award. She holds fifty-eight Honoris Causa doctoral degrees. She received the Department of Defense Legion of Merit Medal, the Smithsonian Institution-James Smithson Bicentennial Medal, the National Governor's Association Distinguished Service to State Government Award during September 11, the YWCA Racial Justice Award, the AMA Board of Trustees Special Award for Meritorious Service, and COSSMHO Humanitarian Award for Lifetime Achievement.

She also won the Congressional Hispanic Caucus Medal; Luther Terry Award for Exemplary Leadership in Tobacco Control; the Charles C. Shepard Science Award for Scientific Excellence; the Nathan Davis Award from the AMA; Hopkins Alumni Association Woodrow Wilson Award for Distinguished Government Service;

the Health Leader Award from the USPHS, Commissioned Officers Association; the Excellence in Crisis and Risk Communication Award from University of Central Florida; the Legacy Award for Science, Smithsonian Institution Latino Center; and the Leadership Award from the Hispanic Heritage Awards, Kennedy Center.

In 1994, she was inducted into the National Women's Hall of Fame (Seneca Falls, New York); in 1996, into the Miami Children's Hospital International Pediatrics Hall of Fame; and in 1990, into the International Women in Medicine Hall of Fame (American Medical Women Association). In 2020 she was listed as one of the one hundred women of the century in commemoration of the 19th amendment and one of the one hundred American women who changed the world. In 2022 the University of Oklahoma School of Medicine honored Dr. Novello as the 2022 Module Renaming Honoree, and the United States Hispanic Leadership Institute established the Antonia Novello Humanitarian Award honoring her service to humanity. Currently she serves as a health advocate of multiple initiatives helping to strengthen trust, knowledge, and participation in current areas of public health.

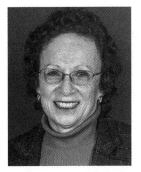

Jill S. Tietjen is the President and CEO of Technically Speaking, Inc. An electrical engineer, she has spent more than forty-five years in the electric utility industry where she provided planning consulting services to electric utilities and organizations comprising the electric utility industry and served as an expert witness before public utility commissions and other government agencies. In 2015, she served as the CEO of the National Women's Hall of Fame, based in Seneca Falls, New York (the birthplace of women's rights). Today, she is a worldwide advocate for telling women's stories and writing women into history.

An author (fourteen books published to date) and international speaker, Tietjen is the co-author of the award-winning and bestselling books *Her Story: A Timeline of the Women Who Changed America* and *Hollywood: Her Story, An Illustrated History of Women and the Movies.* Her latest award-winning book (2022) is *Over, Under, Around, and Through: How Hall of Famers Surmount Obstacles.* Her introduction to engineering textbook, *Keys to Engineering Success,* was published by Prentice Hall in 2001. Her ebook for the Institute of Electrical and Electronics Engineers' Women in Engineering series titled *Recognizing and Taking Advantage of Opportunities* was published in 2016. She is the series editor for Springer's Women in Engineering and Science series, has written two volumes in the series, and has served as co-volume editor for three volumes. She blogged for *The Huffington Post* from 2014 to 2018.

Tietjen has received numerous awards and honors including Women eNews 21 Leaders of the 21st Century (2016); the 2001 Woman in Technology Award from the Women's Foundation of Colorado, Subaru, and News4; Tau Beta Pi's Distinguished Alumna Award; and she was named a Woman of Distinction by Girl Scouts— Mile Hi Council. In 2017, she received the Advocate for Women and Girls Award from Girl Scouts of Colorado and the General Palmer Award from ACEC-Colorado. She served as the 1991–1992 National President of the Society of Women Engineers (SWE). She was the first woman president of the Rocky Mountain Electrical League, the trade association in the West serving the electric utility industry. Tietjen is a member of the Board of Directors for Georgia Transmission Corporation of Tucker, Georgia, and served as an outside director for Merrick & Company of Greenwood Village, Colorado, from 2010 to 2021. She has been inducted into the Colorado Women's Hall of Fame, the Colorado Authors' Hall of Fame, and the National

Academy of Construction. Her story, titled "Engineering Women Back into History," was aired on Rocky Mountain PBS as part of the *Great Colorado Women* film series and is accessible through the Colorado Women's Hall of Fame website film library.

Tietjen graduated from the University of Virginia (Tau Beta Pi, Virginia Alpha) with a BS in Applied Mathematics (minor in Electrical Engineering) and received her MBA from the University of North Carolina–Charlotte. She is a registered professional engineer in Colorado.